A TOOLKIT FOR YOUR EMOTIONS

45 WAYS TO FEEL BETTER

Dr Emma Hepburn
@thepsychologymum

greenfinch

Contents

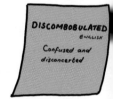

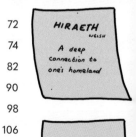

SISU
FINNISH

Extraordinary
determination
in the face of
adversity

FERNWEH
GERMAN

Call of
faraway
places

FEIERABEND
GERMAN

Festive mood
at the end
of a working
day

Your Brain & Emotions

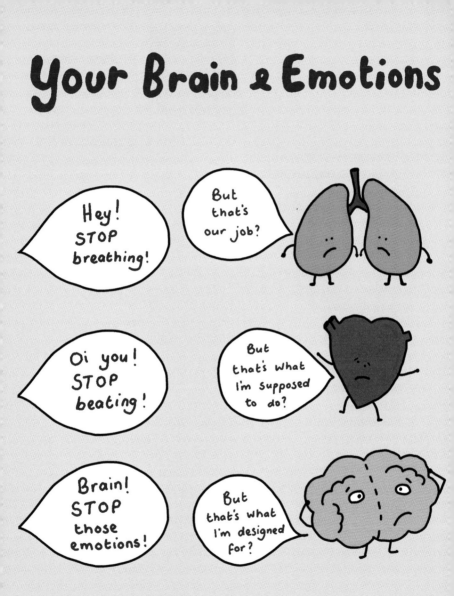

Introduction:
An Emotional World

We all have a lot of emotions during our lives. Personally, I have even had a lot of emotions *about* emotions. For most of my adult life, I have spent a lot of time thinking about emotions – not just as part of my clinical work as a psychologist, but also through my research, lectures and treatment programmes. Here are just a few examples of the emotions about emotions I have felt in my life – perhaps some will resonate with you.

Empathy: Often people see a psychologist when their emotions are getting in the way of life: making them feel bad; stopping them from doing things; or impacting on their health, wellbeing and ability to connect to people. Much of my career has been spent listening to and thinking about emotions – especially the difficult ones that we don't want to speak about – and exploring the stories behind them. The only way to help someone make sense of these emotions is to understand the story that led that person to where they are now. While I listen, my brain creates emotions in me, too. I may feel shock at the stories of trauma, sad at the tales of disappointment and distressed, at times, by experiences beyond my comprehension. Equally, I might feel elated as a small breakthrough comes, when people find themselves climbing out of black holes, experiencing happiness, or connecting to something or someone that makes them feel worthwhile.

Doubt to appreciation: At the start of my clinical psychology journey, I remember feeling doubtful about my emotions. Shouldn't I be able to listen with objectivity? Was it wrong to feel emotions alongside those of others? Then I realized this is simply how our brain is designed – it is human to respond to emotions in others, to understand and empathize. As my career progressed, I started to see my own emotions as beneficial to create connection, to understand the experiences of others, and identify stressors. I now see them as an important part of the therapeutic space. As we'll see in Chapter 1, what we believe about our emotions is important for how we respond and cope. In my case, my beliefs about my own emotions shifted, from frustration to curiosity, acceptance and sometimes appreciation.

Pride (probably misplaced): I haven't always been comfortable with my emotions – like all of us, my own emotions are fundamentally linked to my background, context and beliefs. My children speak freely about emotions. Due to school lessons devised by their brilliant teachers, my children don't think that experiencing emotions makes them weird; it's just something that happens. However, in 1980s Scotland emotions were not part of the school curriculum. My emotional vocabulary was limited to the topics of Norwegian boy bands, reactions to Australian soaps and the films we saw in the cinema. I do remember, though, having pride in how well I could contain big emotions – I was the one who could sit through teenage horror films unscathed (or so I pretended). I fully subscribed to the British idea of a stiff upper lip (ironic for someone who would later become a clinical psychologist and talk about nothing *but* emotions). However, I suspect this was due to the attitudes of the society I grew up in, which was stoic and generally averse to open displays of emotion. None of us can extricate our brain, and its associated emotions, from the context in which it developed and exists. This influences how we perceive, express and respond to our emotions.

Curiosity: I first properly considered emotions during university lectures in my late teens. Before then, I'm not sure if I would have ever thought about what emotions actually are, or if I could have described accurately how I was feeling, beyond the basics of happy, sad or worried. Lectures on emotions and mental health made me feel interested and inspired to see how psychology could be applied to help people with their difficult emotions.

Fascination: After those inspiring lectures, I became so fascinated by emotions that as I came across a new word for an emotion, I collected it, scrawling descriptions on sticky

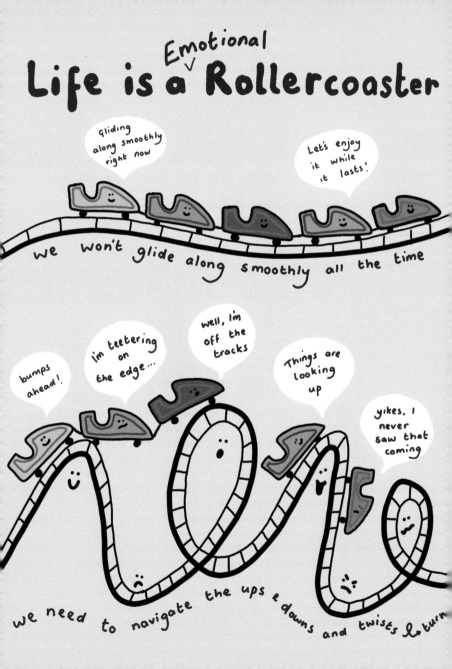

notes and random bills. Sometimes, I even made up words to describe emotions – that bereft feeling when a box set ends, or the joy of having alone time while also missing my children. I stumble across these from time to time and feel nostalgic for my younger self, avidly collecting emotions, not realizing in doing so I was building a vocabulary that would help deepen my understanding and responses to my own emotions, too. You'll find some of my collection scattered through this book on sticky notes. By the time I was working as a clinical psychologist, I felt confident that I knew a lot about emotions: what they were, where they came from, where they existed in the brain. However, little did I know that my emotions about emotions were going to be blown apart.

Discombobulation: Growth in knowledge about the brain in the last decade, has led to big shifts in how we understand emotions. The science of emotions tells us a new story about how they operate in our brain and body (we'll look at this further in Chapter 2). For me, this was discombobulating, as I've had to shift my thinking to incorporate this new knowledge. But that's how science works – new understanding makes us question what we think we know. Overall, it's energizing to consider how this new information might be applied to help people with their emotions.

This book is not about my emotions; it's about everybody's emotions. However, the thing about emotions is they are unique. They are linked to your context, experience and words. They can feel good, bad and all stages in between. They can appear at surprising moments, several at a time, and can be conflicting. They are intrinsically linked to others. But, most importantly, emotions are central to our lives.

This book is the story of emotions, as we cannot tell our own narrative without them. They ride along with us in our lives, directing, diverting, delighting and depressing us. When we look back on our experiences, we don't just remember them, we *feel* them. When we look to our futures, we anticipate how our decisions will make us feel, and our emotions inform those decisions. When we connect to others, we don't just see and hear their stories, we feel them.

Emotions are the central characters in your story, not a single plot point or a byline. They are intrinsic to memory, reactions, future planning, behaviour, connection and ultimately survival. How we understand and respond to our emotions is crucial, and can influence our health and wellbeing across our lifespan. Understanding our emotions can guide us to make decisions compatible with what's important to us, help us deal with the stressors that life throws at us and help us make sense of our lives.

I am sure you will have a lot of emotions while reading this book, as we all have many, every day. Don't dismiss them – take note, and use the exercises in the book to think about them. By doing so, you can start to notice a shift in how you respond to your emotions. As you move forward, you can learn to interact with them differently, or alter your view of what they mean or how you can learn from them. You can learn to build (or create) emotions that support you through life. You can also become better equipped to respond to and navigate the tough emotions, as well as help the feel-good ones stick around for longer. So buckle up, let's go on the rollercoaster ride of the story of emotions, in which *your* emotions will play a starring role.

The emotional rollercoaster

Like all rollercoasters, your emotional rollercoaster will inevitably take you through ups and downs and loop-the-loops as you ride through life. These emotions are an essential, but not always nice, part of life. No two rides are alike, all of us have unique histories, brains and bodies that influence the emotions we experience and how we respond. As you travel through the book, you'll find methods to understand and respond helpfully to your emotions – some of these will feel more relevant to you and some will resonate less.

This image opposite is your emotional rollercoaster, to help you think about what techniques work for you. As you travel through the book, note down your ideas for:
- How you can respond to your emotions.
- What can help you when your rollercoaster dips into tricky emotions.
- Which emotional loop-the-loops you get caught in, and what will help you find routes through these.
- How you can create feel-good emotions, such as calm and joy.
- What tiny tweaks might take your rollercoaster on a new trajectory?

You'll find all of these topics and more in the book, so jot down the ideas that work for you. That way, you can create your own personal travel guide to help you navigate along your emotional rollercoaster.

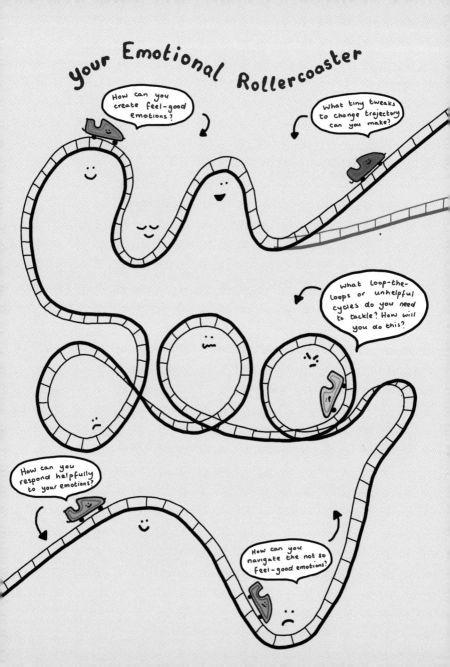

Meet the Emotions

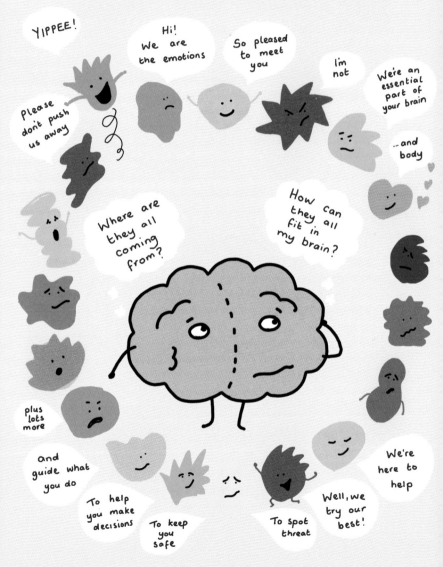

Chapter 1
Getting To Know Emotions

We've all had emotions – our rollercoaster ride takes us through many of them every day. But have you ever stopped to wonder what they really are? What are these things that have so much influence over our lives, and why do we have the ups, downs and loop-the-loops of emotion? These questions are not as easy to answer as you might think. To help answer them (as best as the current science can), we're going to journey to imaginary lands, time travel to the past (briefly stopping to meet Darwin), zoom into the future, and even bake some cookies. You may well experience some emotions as we travel: perhaps relief, as we blast some emotion myths off the track; maybe puzzlement, as we challenge your beliefs about what emotions really are; possibly enjoyment, as we bake some emotion cookies; and hopefully wonder, at your amazing brain and its powerful predictive superpower, which is always one step ahead of you. Of course, you may feel none of these emotions, or you may feel different emotions altogether, because, as we'll find as we travel through this chapter, the possibilities of emotions are as variable as the type and flavour of cookies that exist in the world.

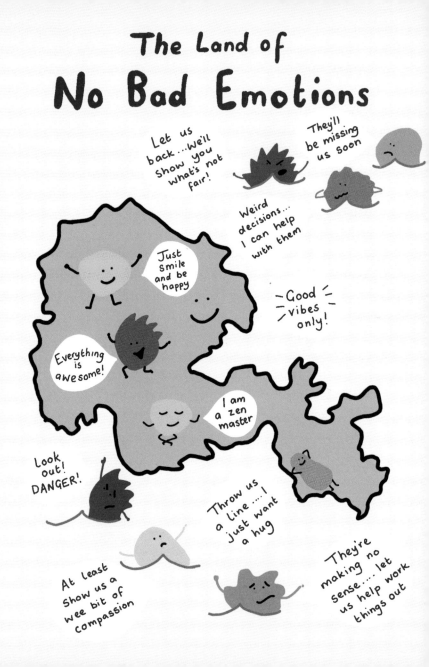

Why do we have emotions?

Before I try to define emotions, let's first think about their purpose. Why do we have feelings that can make us ride that emotional rollercoaster? Yes, emotions sometimes make us feel on top of the world, free-wheeling on joy, but they can also plunge us to the depths of darkness, immobilize us or make us feel out of control. If we could only experience the good ones and get rid of all those horrible ones, wouldn't all our lives be better?

The land of No Bad Emotions

To answer this question, and consider why emotions are central to our lives, let's take a brief detour to the realms of a seemingly utopian world of No Bad Emotions. A place where negative emotions have been banished. Here, people don't feel stress, anger, fear, upset, bitterness, jealousy, guilt or sadness. It's a modern-day pleasure dome of blissful living. Yet, soon the cracks start to appear. There's something odd about the decision-making of inhabitants in our sad-free land. They don't seem to consider risk or the impact of their decisions on themselves or others. They don't seem to learn from past experience to make better decisions.

In fact, the inhabitants are making decisions that are far from what we would consider rational. When threat appears, they don't spot it and take immediate action – they become passive bystanders, inanely watching as these risks might hurt or even kill them. When people die, there's no mourning. When illness strikes, people don't stop and rest. They feel great, so keep going, allowing illness to wreak havoc by giving their bodies no chance to recuperate.

Connections also seem to be breaking down. People don't notice when they've crossed a social boundary, so no apologies or shifts in behaviour are forthcoming. There's no anger when values are transgressed, so no action taken. Inhabitants don't feel compassion for other people's stories; they don't dish out hugs in response to difficulty, or sit with others in empathy. In turn, joy becomes meaningless. With no comparison, it's hard to recognize feeling good. People can no longer differentiate between factors that create delight and danger; they have no incoming sensory data to tell them snakes are dangerous or that rotten tomatoes might poison them. They have no information to tell them what is good or bad for them, or direct them how to best spend their limited time on Earth.

Our emotional utopia slowly turns into a dystopia, because emotions (and not just the feel-good ones) are essential for humans. They support our decision-making and reasoning. They help us process sensory input and give it meaning. They help us understand the world and how to respond. They help us to communicate and empathize. They help our brain predict the future, based on our past experiences. They help us live and survive. Nobody's pretending that our emotions are perfectly designed or always helpful: they often get in the way, and can impact negatively on our actions and decisions. But, if given the option, choosing to have emotions (and all of them) is far better than choosing not to.

We've been making our emotions feel bad for long enough! It's time to give them the credit they deserve by considering just some of the ways they help us get through life.

Emotions help us make sense of our complex world. Every moment of every day we have an overwhelming amount of data coming at us, which the brain needs to make sense of. So, it creates concepts to divide this data into manageable constructs that help us answer questions such as 'What the heck is happening?' and 'What should I do?' Emotions are your brain constructing meaning from all the data, including your body data, to determine what to do. 'What's that furry thing? It's a dog. Okay, I like dogs. No wait, that furry, growling thing – that's a danger. I feel fear...run now!' With the second dog, your brain combined the external data with this internal data (body sensations) to make sense of it, and determined you were fearful and needed to act immediately. Emotions support us to make meaning out of a mass of information and make sense of what is happening.

Emotions support decision-making. Emotions are central to our decisions. Yes, sometimes they might drive us in the wrong direction, but they can also help us build on past knowledge, identify risk and act on it. Emotions researcher Antonio Damasio says, 'Well deployed emotions appear to be a support system without which...reason cannot operate properly.' Emotions can also help identify problems. They can signal that something needs to change or something is creating stress that we need to problem-solve.

Emotions are not irrational. The man-made battle between emotions and rationality goes as far back as Plato hypothesizing in ancient Greece. For centuries, reason has been seen as a superior human ability doing battle with unreasonable emotions. Versions of this story are told in many ways: morality versus immorality; rationality versus irrationality; instinct versus self-restraint. This plays out today in psychology books that talk about three brain layers: a lizard brain responsible for basic instincts; a monkey or mammalian brain responsible for emotions; and our uniquely human neocortex, responsible for rationality and reasoning, which keeps the other parts in check. Let's be clear – if anybody tells you that you have a lizard in your brain, don't believe them. The basic brain anatomy behind this idea is flawed, as it's not based on how our brains evolved or work. Emotions and rationality do not sit in separate parts of the brain at odds with each other; they are intrinsically intertwined. If we think about it, emotions are often perfectly rational. Feeling threatened when someone shouts at you in the street, or feeling sad when your much-loved goldfish dies – both are very rational. Even emotions that seem totally illogical at a particular moment can make sense if we look at where they came from.

Emotions help us stay safe and survive. Without emotions, we wouldn't feel fear when necessary and would probably get bitten by that second dog we saw earlier (see page 21). Emotions help us spot the risks emerging from the mass of data coming at us and use our experiences to predict risk, to know what to run away from. They put our body and mind in states that help us manage that risk, and ultimately keep us alive.

Emotions are tied intrinsically to memory. Think back to an unhappy time in your life: you will not just recall images or words, you will *feel* those memories. How we feel is an intrinsic part of memories, and these guide our actions in the present, telling us what to expect from the current situation based on what we learned about it last time. To make sense of current information, our brain checks for data from its data bank that best matches it and reacts accordingly.

Emotions help us know what actions to take (by helping us predict the future). From the above examples, we can see that how we feel helps identify what we need to do in the situation in which we find ourselves. This might be an action of behaviour, such as crying at a sad film or hiding from a scary dog. Or you might feel grumpy because you're hungry and need to eat quickly. Emotions are signals that help our brain direct our physical responses, and take action if needed. This is useful when you've forgotten to have lunch, or there is a threat you need to respond to, but your brain sometimes continues to apply rules or make predictions when they are no longer relevant. Understanding why these responses are created gives us vital tools to intercept them.

Emotions help us manage our resources. One of the key reasons for emotions (and a primary purpose for our brain, as it turns out) is to help manage our 'body budget'. We have limited energy and resources, and our brain needs to manage these wisely. In fact, energy has historically been associated with emotions; the word 'emotion' derives from *mot* (the Latin word for movement) and came to be used in Britain in the 17th century, when it was used to describe bodily movements. This evolved in the 18th century to describe bodily movements or changes associated with mental feelings (see Further Reading on page 188 for more information). Emotions (for example, nervousness) direct your brain to tell your body what it needs to do to help you. Does your body need to send more energy to your brain to make it alert because the person approaching is your manager, or can you save energy and relax because it's actually your friend? How you feel at any point in time can help you and your brain make decisions about when to expend energy and when it's okay to conserve it. Your brain is constantly working away in the background to try and manage energy deposits and withdrawals to maintain a healthy equilibrium.

Emotions help us to connect with others. Emotions provide a culturally common language that helps us convey meaning, connect with others and lets others understand how to respond. Our brain is also constantly perceiving how others feel and reacting to this with our own feelings, so it can know what action to take. A distressing newsreel prompts you to donate; a hug for your upset child helps calm their – and your – nervous system. Emotions bond us together, interconnecting our brains and bodies, and enabling us to support others and help them thrive.

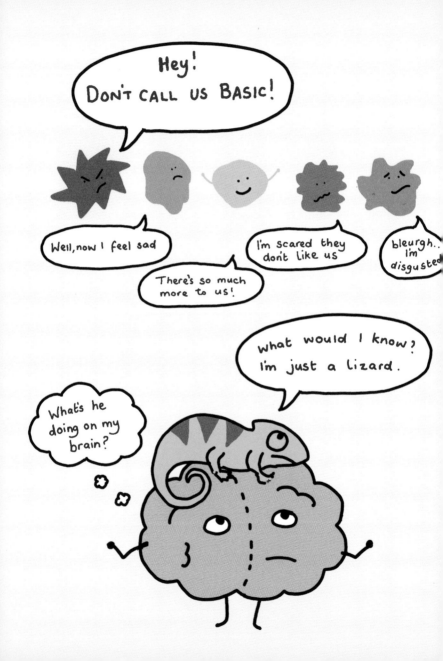

Don't call us basic

Emotions may rightly feel a little disgruntled at how they've been treated over the course of history. They've been described as irrational responses or troubling desires and passions. They've even been entirely neglected, as the word 'emotion' didn't exist as we use it today until the early 19th century, when Scottish Professor of Moral Philosophy Thomas Brown proposed we should study emotions as a scientific category. Of course, it's not that we didn't have emotions before then, it's just that we didn't describe them as such. Getting a name (finally) wasn't the end of the matter. Since then, people have struggled to define emotions. They've been misunderstood, described as shameful or something negative that you shouldn't experience. People say emotions are all in the mind. They've been viewed as unwanted or unnecessary. And it's perhaps not the worst insult thrown at them, but they've also been called 'basic'.

Are emotions really basic?

I learned the idea of basic, or universal, emotions at university, and I accepted it without question. A simplified version goes something like this: our brains are wired to have a set of common emotions that we all share regardless of who or where we are and in which culture we live. Each of these emotions has a distinct physiological response in our brain and body and we can spot the specific emotion through the associated signs, be that brain patterns, facial expression, physical signs or behaviour. Essentially, each basic emotion has a blueprint of brain and body reactions, and these are triggered by whatever is happening in our life. They are universal because we all have them.

This idea has roots in the theories of evolutionary whizz-kid Charles Darwin. He considered emotions within the context of evolution – how did they serve us? Well, there are many ways: love helps us connect, produce and protect our young, ultimately helping us survive. Anger helps us protect our territory, protect our loved ones and (again) survive. Darwin's book *The Expression of the Emotions in Man and Animals*, published in 1872, seemed to confirm the then widely-held view that we have a number of basic emotions, each associated with specific triggers and brain structures, and which result in specific behaviours. Travel forward to 1977 and Carl Sagan popularized the idea of the 'triune brain' (originally proposed by neuroscientist Paul MacLean in 1969): the evolutionary brain model that evolved in ever more sophisticated stages from primitive lizard, to emotional, to rational brain (see also page 22). This perpetuated the age-old idea that our brain has specific emotion regions, which are in a tug-of-war with more sophisticated rational regions.

This idea of universal and basic emotions powerfully pervaded our emotional psyche and culture up until the

1990s and beyond. Research seemed to back it up: Paul Ekman's studies showed pictures of facial expressions to people across the world who reliably matched them to emotion words. While the amount of universal emotions has been debated (and varies in different theories from 4 to 27 or more), there appeared to be a general consensus that we had pinned down how emotions work. Each emotion has a predictable physiological and brain pattern that defines and differentiates it. This view is still commonly held. Many textbooks in university libraries argue in favour of this theory today. You will also find this notion influencing aspects of popular culture. Have you ever seen the children's film *Inside Out*? It's a wonderful depiction of how emotions affect our lives. Watch closely and you'll see the characters are based on basic emotions, existing in discrete categories in our brain. While some emotional patterns are common, there is no evidence to suggest that they originate in specific regions of the brain, nor can any emotion be as clear cut and simple as the theory suggests.

The theory of constructed emotions

It turns out it can be hard to define emotions generally. If you ask several people what emotions are, you'll get a range of views. This question is probably not as simple as it first appears, as there is no universally agreed answer. How to define exactly what emotions are is a topic of huge debate. In fact, 92 different definitions have been found in current research. So, emotions probably shouldn't be called basic. To find out why, we need to look at some of the most recent research. And it all starts with failure.

I imagine Lisa Feldman-Barrett felt dejected when her initial psychological experiments appeared to be failing. Why could her participants not distinguish clearly between what should be distinct emotions of anxiety and depression? Why could she not find and differentiate clear physical responses of different emotions? Her research looked at brain activity, facial expression and body activity during thousands of incidents of emotion and found no consistent pattern associated with specific emotion categories. Feldman-Barrett's work has also questioned whether it is possible to universally name emotions across cultures. Her research has called into question the very nature of emotions. They are not simply a reaction to what's going on around us: but something that our brain actively constructs to help us understand the world in which we live. This is our new understanding – the theory of 'constructed emotions'.

Brain research has evolved remarkably in the last few decades – it has dispelled that lizard from our brain and shown there is no standard pattern for each emotion. How one person experiences an emotion is likely to differ markedly in their description, subjective experience and brain and body activity from others. While our brains may all look similar, the connections in them are as infinitely variable as people, meaning variation is the norm for how they work and for how we experience emotions.

We now know that our brain is an active participant in building our emotions, using its understanding of data to create meaning. Our brain creates emotions by using its past knowledge of the world to combine our internal data (body sensations) with the external data (context) to give them meaning and guide our actions. Taking time to understand how your brain constructs emotions has important implications for how we understand ourselves – and what it means to be human. It also puts more power in your hands to influence how you feel on a daily basis: instead of being surprised and terrified on your emotional rollercoaster, I want to show you how to spot the twists and turns and be able to ride out even the really challenging emotions we all face.

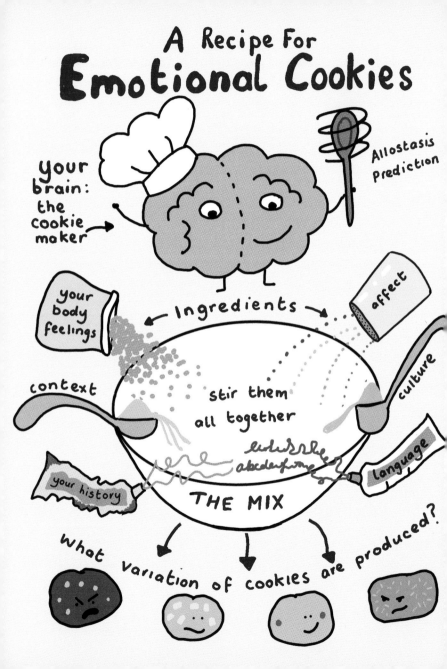

A recipe for emotions

Current neuroscience suggests we make our emotions, but here, we are going to *bake* them! Baking emotional cookies is an analogy used by Lisa Feldman-Barrett that I think captures nicely why our emotions differ so much across people, places and times. To me, viewing our emotions as cookies makes them a lot friendlier and more manageable. Sometimes they might taste wonderful, other times not so good, but ultimately they are there to sustain us. The bake might go wrong, but we can learn from this and tweak the ingredients to make them a bit different next time.

Although the ingredients in cookies look fairly standard, they are not the same for all. There is much variation in what these ingredients look like in real life, which means we all have a different dough and will never end up with the same emotional cookies. Tweak one ingredient (you might be feeling more tired, for example) and what goes into the bake differs, along with the outcome. There are infinite possibilities and outcomes, because the ingredients are endlessly variable – be that our brain, experiences or body. So, let's start baking some emotional cookies!

The cookie maker

Before we look at our ingredients, let's consider the cookie maker that combines all the ingredients to create the final output of an emotion – your brain. It's the head chef, working in the kitchen making sense of everything coming in, and working out what it needs to do in response. So, we need to understand some of the functions your brain performs that are central to combining the cookie mix.

Allostasis: In order to maintain the body's energy budget (that we covered on page 24) the brain needs to predict energy needs before they happen, so it can respond effectively – this process is called 'allostasis'. Your brain anticipates when you need energy to run away from that scary thing, when it needs to rest and when it needs an energy boost (a double latte for me, please). Predictions are at the heart of allostasis, because they enable your brain to direct its resources where necessary and get your body ready to respond appropriately to what's coming your way. This creates body sensations, which contribute to emotions. But in order to make these predictions, your brain needs the first ingredient...

Ingredients for your emotional cookies
Ingredient 1: **Your history**
How does this amazing future-focused organ of ours create its predictions? Well, it bases its best guess of what is about to happen on what it knows already – the past. Your past has helped wire your brain's networks to understand your world. Your brain matches the information coming at it with the

most similar and salient existing information in its knowledge stores, and this tells the brain how it needs to react. You're sitting outside in the sun relaxing with a smoothie when your eye catches a glimpse of something flying past; your brain checks its information bank and its best guess is a malevolent wasp, with your sweet drink as its most likely target. Your brain prepares your body for action, to swat the wasp or move your drink. You look again, see a flash of red, and your brain re-categorizes the wasp to a gentle ladybird, telling your body to enjoy the experience instead. This process also helps categorize emotions, as your brain matches what you are experiencing in that context to the closest match from its memory bank, to help define which emotion you are experiencing.

Ingredient 2: Your body

Your body is constantly performing a multitude of functions to keep you alive. Some you will be aware of (your grumbling stomach or the increased heart rate when you see that wasp), but many you won't (your immune responses constantly alert to fight invaders to your body or your neurons linking together creating connections in your brain). All day, every day, your complex body systems are working overtime to support you – and your brain is the master in the control room, keeping the factory functioning, with regular subtle tweaks in response to feedback it's getting. Not all of this will come into your awareness, but when it does, your brain makes sense of these body sensations using the context of the outside world. In our example, when you saw a wasp, your brain understood what was happening through a combination of looking at the external and internal data, as an instance of fear. However, the same body sensation in a different context, for example in a crowd at a concert, might be thought of as excitement (unless you hate crowds, in which case you might understand this as fear). Our body sensations help us understand what is going on in a given situation, and are a key ingredient in our emotions.

Ingredient 3: **Mood (or affect)**

Our mood (or being scientific, our 'affect') is our general sense of how we are feeling – the 'bleurgh', the 'meh' and the 'yay' of our day are important parts of the emotions mix. Hunger, thirst, illness, your temperature, brain chemicals, hormones, organ functioning, who we are with, how much energy we've used, how tired we are – these body processes (and many more) all contribute to how we feel at any given moment. After all, mood is your brain's clever way of summarizing all that is going on in your body. Feldman-Barrett describes affect as like 'a barometer for how you are doing...affect hints whether your body budget is in balance or in the red'. To me, affect demonstrates why it makes no sense to divide the body and mind, as they work intrinsically together. All the physical processes are summarized by our mood – a general indicator that you feel either bad or good.

Mood is the universal bedrock of feelings that we all experience, and varies along two dimensions: arousal (high energy or low energy); and valence (pleasant or unpleasant).

Ingredient 4: **Your context**

We've already alluded to this ingredient a number of times, but sometimes it's so obvious it gets missed out of the mix. Your context is the external data that is coming at you on a regular basis and which impacts on your predictions and body budget. Are you experiencing daily threats, which your brain has to respond to by getting your body revved up? Do you feel safe, which enables your body budget to conserve and replenish? Do the people around you regulate your nervous system and help your body keep itself in balance, or do they throw it out of kilter? Your daily context is also crucial for how your brain decides to best categorize the emotion you're feeling. As we've seen, the same physical sensations in different contexts may be defined differently – excited at a concert or nervous before an exam, for example.

Ingredient 5: **Your culture**

Our emotions are constructed using the knowledge structure in our brain, and those structures and concepts are intrinsically linked to our cultural background. We could even say emotions are cultural. How we respond to grief, what we perceive sadness should look like (if we perceive sadness at all), what we even think about emotions are all linked to the culture in which we exist. In fact, the word emotion doesn't even exist in some cultures. So, what we feel, how we feel it and how we respond to this is enmeshed with the ideas of our culture. Our beliefs also help create our emotions, as they influence what our brains predict and how our bodies respond in different situations – what we think we should do when grieving, for example, will inform what our body and brain do in this situation. Will we scream or cry silently? We create and share our collective understanding of these concepts and categorize these through language, which brings us nicely to our last ingredient…

Ingredient 6: Your language

Language is the tool we use to label, categorize and understand the world. Happiness, anxiety, frustration, anger are all linguistic labels to categorize and understand our emotions and to communicate this to others. The words we use to describe how we feel help us make sense of these feelings and decide what to do about them. They provide structure and meaning to our complex sensory, external and internal input. We might assume with emotions that one label (e.g. anger) equals one thing. However, labels tend to categorize a range of similar things under one concept, and this is the same for the language of emotions. A dog could mean a pit bull, a cockapoo or a great dane. This is exactly the same for emotion concepts. Anger is a broad category, and might mean being furious because of a grave miscarriage of justice, or feeling undermined when someone has belittled you in a meeting. How you feel for each of these incidents may vary from tears to blushing, to full-on shouting. Each emotion category is defined by variation and includes a range of possible experiences, feelings, body reactions and behaviours, which will differ between people and situations.

Infinite recipes

When we take the emotion cookies out of the oven, the end results will vary between different people and even at different times for the same person, because there are so many possible ingredients and cookie mixes. Emotions are our brain's attempt to understand how we feel, by categorizing and giving concepts to a complex mix of incoming internal and external data, ultimately in order to help us survive and thrive. There may be a few common ingredients that create these emotions, but these result in an infinite number of variations in the end result.

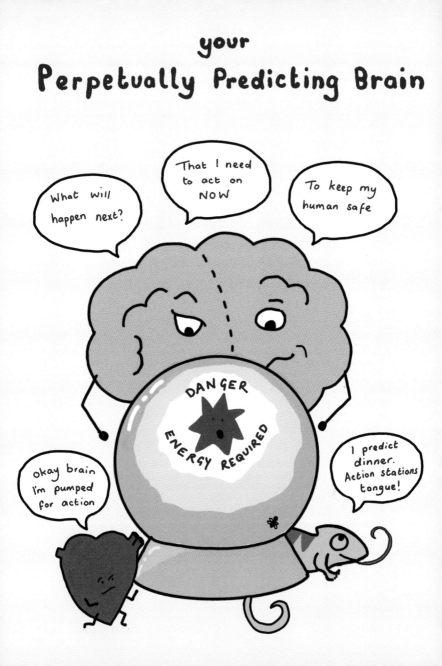

I predict a riot!

Emotions are not reactions; they are constructions of what a body sensation means in a particular context. Does this mean we are to blame for our emotions? Definitely not. Our brain's understanding, and indeed the body responses themselves, are created based on past experience, and we can't change that, nor how we feel in the moment. However, if we start to see ourselves as the architect of emotions, rather than our emotions being uncontrollable reactions, we can help our brain learn to predict and respond differently. We can look to the future to think where we want our rollercoaster to go, guide it and understand why, despite our best efforts, it sometimes gets stuck in a dip. Understanding why our brain is doing what it is doing also allows us to better tolerate the inevitable emotions we experience. So, let's get to know your brain and the body it exists in a bit better.

Your brain's superpower

Neuroscientist Karl Friston described the brain as 'an organ of prediction driving a vulnerable body through an uncertain world'. In fact, prediction could be considered your brain's superpower, as it is perpetually using every second and every minute of the day to anticipate what will happen next, getting your body ready to respond. These predictions are at the heart of allostasis (see page 34), because they enable your brain to direct its resources as it sees fit for what it predicts is about to come. Your brain is always one step ahead of you – even reading this now, it is predicting the next coffee. Okay, I meant to end that sentence with 'word', as that is what your brain will most likely have predicted (unless you are desperate for a caffeine fix). Perhaps reading it created a small moment of surprise as your brain quickly had to adjust to recognize its prediction was wrong? A powerful prediction experience is when you walk up a broken escalator and it feels like it's still moving, because your brain is predicting it will move. In fact, much of the world we experience is based on our brains' predictions.

These predictions are your brain's best quick-fire guesses of what will happen in the next moment, based on the knowledge base you have built up through your life. This allows us to be one step ahead of reality. If our brain decided how to react only after a thorough factual analysis of each situation, we would not survive as a species – we would be too slow to react to danger. If your predictions tell your brain it needs more energy, your brain starts to rev up your body to enable it to take timely action. It's this body response that feeds into how we feel. Not all body sensations are understood as emotions, of course – some of the body sensations we experience tell us we are hungry, for example. If you are sensitive to low blood sugar, you might also experience this as an emotion such as feeling grumpy, or 'hangry'. Our brain's predictive powers are at work when we anticipate eating, and our hunger satiates well before the food has had a chance to break down and release energy through our body. If you experience hanger, then you may have wondered why you feel better as soon as you bite into food? Your brain has predicted that you should now feel okay and has adjusted your body response immediately.

However, sometimes the predictions that our brain issues are not so helpful. For example, just as I am getting ready for sleep after a hard day's work, my brain seems to wake me up and I'm no longer tired. To understand this response, we need to delve into my past. I've never been good at getting to sleep. Many factors play into this – my physiology makes me a night owl who would work until two in the morning and wake up later. However, this doesn't fit with school or work, so I've had to try to get to sleep earlier throughout my life. I spent many hours during my teens and twenties lying awake not able to sleep, which is not the most pleasant experience. As a result, when my brain now thinks of bed, instead of relaxing me, it gets my body revved up to deal with this predicted difficulty getting to sleep. Thank you very much, brain – this is not helpful. Over the years, I have taught my brain to stop predicting difficulty at bedtime by creating a relaxing and enjoyable bedtime routine it can look forward to instead.

I predict the future

If you had a bad boss in the past, no matter how nice your next boss is, your brain will continue to issue predictions that you need to get ready for action to deal with the threat when you meet with your boss. It will take time to correct these predictions, so that you start to look forward to the meetings with your caring boss. If you have been through chronic stressors, your brain will be issuing predictions that you need to be on high alert to get ready to deal with the next imminent stressor. It can take a while for your brain to correct this prediction after the stressful period has passed, so it continues to put you on high alert when this response is no longer required (over-predicting rather than under-predicting threat ultimately keeps us safe). This explains partly why our emotions are not always related objectively to what's going on in the current environment – the brain continues to issue predictions even after the event, which can be unhelpful when they no longer fit with our current context.

We might wonder why something creates anxiety in one person, when it makes another feel safe and secure? Why is one person's cute, cuddly rat another person's terror? Well, different brains issue different predictions for the current data depending on the knowledge structures they hold. These different predictions make our bodies respond in different ways, which impacts how we feel. As we saw in our emotional cookies (page 32), predictions aren't the whole story (in the next chapter we'll look at other factors that impact on our body and feed into our moods). However, the predictions our brain makes, and why it makes them, are important parts of our emotional rollercoaster, constantly driving it forward. While you might think you are riding along in the moment enjoying the ride, your brain is always one step ahead, predicting what's around the corner and how to best use your body budget to help you survive.

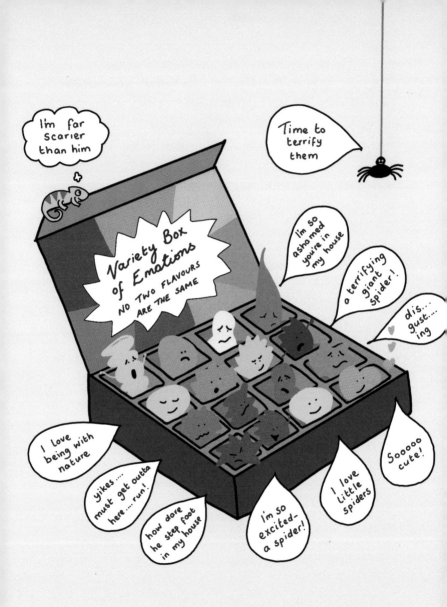

Chapter 2
Why We All React Differently

You might hope that your emotional rollercoaster will take you on a smooth ride through life, with very few ups and downs. This is possible, but highly unlikely. Each of our lives will throw different things at us, and we all have to navigate an unpredictable world. It's much more likely that your rollercoaster will travel through ups and downs, loop-the-loops, spirals and maybe even into dark tunnels out of which you have to navigate your way. Each of our rollercoasters will look different, take different turns and follow different paths. We all have different minds, bodies and experiences, which means that how our brains predict, understand and respond to our lives will vary. This chapter looks at understanding some of the factors that feed into your unique emotional journey and starts to explore how we can help navigate some of the inevitable challenges life flings at us along the route.

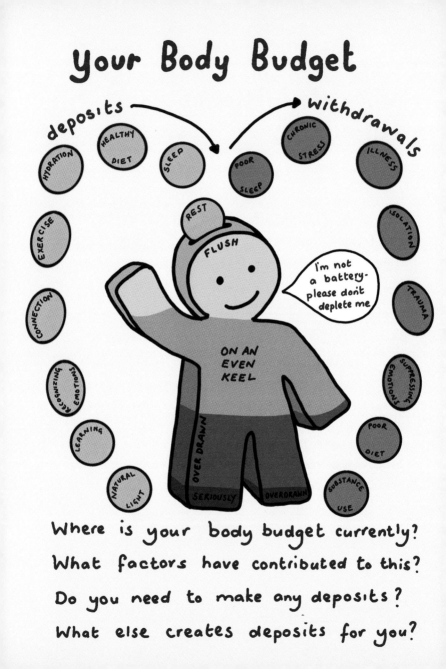

Your Body Budget

Where is your body budget currently?
What factors have contributed to this?
Do you need to make any deposits?
What else creates deposits for you?

A variety box of emotions

If we put twenty people in a room with spiders, their body and brain responses and emotional experiences would vary. Even two people who describe a similar emotion, such as feeling scared, might have very different body and brain responses. When my children see a spider and I tell them, 'There's nothing to be scared of', I am factually incorrect. *My brain* may not be creating a body sensation that's understood as fear, but if *their brains* are predicting differently, creating a body response that they understand as fear, that is entirely real and valid. So, my response is dismissive of the emotion they are experiencing. Sorry, kids!

We might think we should be able to look at objects or events and determine an objective reaction. The correct response for a burglar would be fear, while a butterfly provokes wonder, for example. However, it's not that easy, and the myth that people should be feeling a certain way in a particular situation can contribute to emotional and mental-health stigma. We've all heard variations of 'You should be happy, look how lucky you are', 'What's he got to be sad about?' or my own 'There's nothing to be scared of'. We apply these maxims to ourselves and others, leading us to think that how we are feeling is 'wrong' in some way (which can lead to greater negative emotions, as we'll see in Chapter 3). However, in doing so, we fail to recognize that each individual's background and experience is unique. You cannot say how someone should or will feel, so let's stop using that as a stick to beat ourselves or other people.

Based on those pretty pictures of brain scans so common nowadays, you might think that we all have similar brains that work in the same ways. It's true that if we look inside, there are usually (but not always) similar structures, and we can predict (to some extent) that damage to certain areas will impact on particular functions. But structure is just part of the picture, and it gets more interesting when we start thinking about connections. We have around 85 billion neurons in our brain, which connect to one another through electrical impulses, supported by chemicals – neurotransmitters and neuromodulators. Not all neurons connect, but the ones that do create a mindboggling number of connections – around 500 trillion. Complex networks link areas of our brain (which link to our body, too). Each neuron has a range of purposes, and different groups of neurons can achieve the same purpose (a process called 'degeneracy'), meaning the possible patterns of connections are vast, flexible and changeable. Although all our brains work in the same general way, each brain 'tunes and prunes to its surroundings'. This means your connections are yours and yours alone.

It's quite incredible to think no one else in the entire world has a mind just like yours, or no two brains function in exactly the same way. Our complex brain adapts and wires itself to the environment in which it exists. As you grow, learn and proceed through life, your brain encodes and creates patterns to account for the information that comes your way and uses this to understand and predict future information. Your 85 billions neurons, alongside supporting structures and chemicals, can never work in exactly the same way as anyone else's. That's why it makes no sense to compare how you respond in any given situation to anyone else; you are not the same, your minds work differently. Of course, there is some commonality of human experience, and tendencies (especially within cultures) to react to situations in particular ways. This collective understanding of our experiences can help validate how we feel on an individual level. However, each response remains unique across a range of variables. It is helpful to seek commonalities for our benefit but not disparage the differences to our detriment.

Of course, your brain and body are not separate, they are in perpetual conversation – your brain is part of your body, and your brain and body help create your mind. We've seen already that your brain aims to makes sense of body sensations, and some of this results in emotions. What goes on in your body is part of creating emotions and results in that summary of your body budget – affect. Just like the mind, all individual bodies function slightly differently, producing different data and affect for our brains to interpret. These differences can range across many body mechanisms: control of blood sugar levels; how fast our heart beats; how our immune system functions; experience of pain; how our muscles respond; what's going on in our gut, etc. There is so much variation in how our individual bodies function and what impacts on this that it should be no surprise that the data that contributes to how we feel is vast, and changes across individuals and between the same individual on different days.

Our recent experiences, too, impact on what's going on in our body – how we slept last night, how much stress we are under, whether we've exercised, what we've eaten and more. Your brain is constantly trying to keep your body budget in balance – we can think of this as withdrawals and deposits. Your body budget fluctuates throughout the day and you can get it back into a positive balance with deposits such as rest and sleep. However, too many withdrawals, for example due to stress or when your brain wrongly predicts your body energy needs over a long period of time, can leave your budget severely overdrawn and in the red. All this impacts on how you feel and your affect. This is why looking after your body is such a crucial part of looking after your emotions.

One commonality of human experience is thought to be affect or mood – that general sense of whether you are feeling good that comes from your body. Even though the experience of affect is collective, our introspection and experience of sensations also differs. Some people are finely attuned to their body and notice subtle changes; others are less aware. Our attention at times may be more directed to notice our body sensation or affect due to our experiences (if you've ever had a health scare, you'll find you're suddenly much more likely to notice body sensations). Our affect can also be variable – some people's mood fluctuates wildly, while others appear to breeze along in a sea of calm. And, of course, what makes us feel different affect varies widely. Some people are hypersensitive to what's going on around them and are affected by others' emotions, while some are more self-contained.

Once we accept that variation is the norm when it comes to emotions, we can start to understand and notice some of the components that contribute to the range of emotions we will experience over our lifetime. Understanding these can help us to work with these building blocks to respond differently to our needs and build different emotions on our emotional rollercoaster.

Notice your body budget

Use the image and questions on page 48 to help you work out where your current body budget is. Are you flush because you have just come back from a relaxing break, or are you in the red because you are in the middle of high stress? Try using a mental body scan, which means working through your body in your mind, from head to toe, to see what's going on. Ask yourself how you are feeling a few times a day, so you can begin to listen to what your body is telling you. Think about what you are feeling and how you would summarize your body budget.

Managing your body budget

We are constantly making withdrawals from and deposits to our body budget, and these are important for affect and emotions. Sometimes we fail to notice when deposits are required, or dismiss the importance of them. Sometimes we make temporary deposits, such as caffeine or alcohol, which top our body up briefly but mask the underlying depletion of resources. Use the checklist here and the image on page 48 to consider what withdrawals are currently happening in your life and how you can make deposits when you need to. Many of the things that create deposits may seem basic, but that's exactly why we overlook them and their impact on not just our body, but also our emotions through how we feel.

Deposits:

- ☐ Sleep
- ☐ Rest
- ☐ Eating well
- ☐ Hydration
- ☐ Exercise/ movement
- ☐ Positive social connections
- ☐ Recognizing emotions
- ☐ Natural light
- ☐ Learning
- ☐ Being in nature
- ☐ Fun and laughter
- ☐ Physical comfort
- ☐ Cuddles
- ☐ Being creative

Withdrawals:

- ☐ Chronic stress
- ☐ Poor sleep
- ☐ Poor diet
- ☐ Illness
- ☐ Pain
- ☐ Social isolation
- ☐ Lack of exercise/ movement
- ☐ Suppressing emotions
- ☐ Substance use
- ☐ Excessive tech/phone use
- ☐ Lack of rest
- ☐ Trauma
- ☐ Overwork

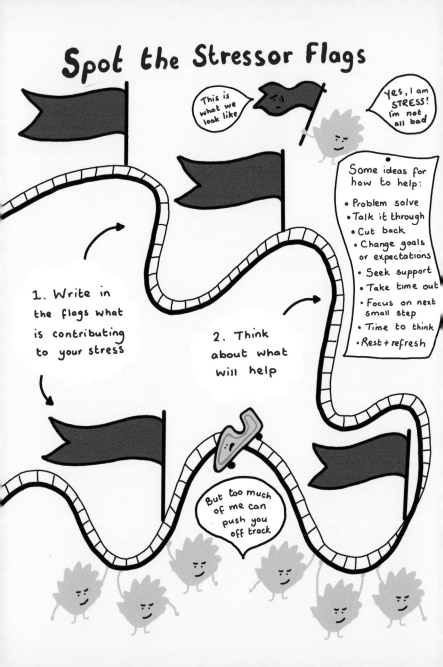

The world around us

We are all navigating an unpredictable world on our emotional rollercoaster. Humans like predictability, and our brain is designed to find meaning and patterns in the data coming our way. Greater predictability helps conserve our resources and helps us survive. However, no matter how organized we are (which is essentially us predicting our day-to-day world), uncertainty will come our way. This impacts our brain and body budget – it's demanding for our brain to deal with situations that are difficult to predict. If the data coming at our brain does not align with its predictions, it needs to regroup, try to understand and correct its prediction. Uncertainty over what is happening next means our brain is likely to predict that it needs to get revved up to respond to whatever is coming its way, and that uses energy. It requires a lot of cognitive resources to respond to uncertainty, which is also metabolically demanding and creates withdrawals from our body budget. If this goes on for too long we can become depleted, suffering from an overdrawn body budget that leads to burnout and all manner of health difficulties.

Never has this been so apparent than during the Covid-19 pandemic. Years of uncertainty (both health and economic), constantly shifting to live under new rules, as well as having to understand concepts we'd never heard of previously has impacted on our body budgets. It's no wonder that so many people are feeling burnt out or exhausted.

Unpredictable threats come in different forms. That bullying boss, the undermining family member, the child who has no sense of danger of passing traffic, the pavement not designed for wheelchair users – all require vigilance from your brain. Any situation where you feel unsafe (bullying, racism, discrimination or harassment, for example) means your brain is predicting threat and needs to be pumped up, placing demands on your body budget. We also know that if you were brought up feeling unsafe, your brain will wire itself to this context, creating patterns designed to protect you from harm but which may not always help as you grow older.

So far, I've touched on what could be described as negative 'stressors' – an inevitable part of the emotional rollercoaster ride, and of life. However, stressors can be both positive and negative – being on a real-life fairground rollercoaster causes your heart to race, and a physically and mentally revved-up state that might be a negative experience for some people, but a joyful, life-affirming one for others. Stressors can also be described as acute (short term) or chronic (long term). Starting a new job requiring additional learning might be considered an exhilarating and positive stressor. Having an argument with your child might be a negative stressor that is only short term and easy to recover from. When stressed, the brain sets off a chain of reactions commonly called some variation of the 'flight, fight, freeze' response. Your body's sympathetic nervous system releases adrenaline and cortisol to get you ready for action to deal with a stressor. This places demand on your body's budget, but everyday stressors happen to everybody; they are part of life. Often your body can recover from them, and in fact it may even strengthen in response.

Stressors create emotion, but this response won't always be labelled as stress – this is just one emotional label we can apply to understand what's going on. The emotions that result from the fight, flight, freeze response can be varied and depend on context. Sometimes the response can be exhilarating, for example if we are exercising or enjoy watching horror films, we may label it as pleasure or excitement. Sometimes it can be scary or anxiety-provoking when it seems to come out of the blue and you feel your heart beating uncontrollably, which we might say is fear. We cannot say exactly which emotion will arise, as it depends on all the other ingredients going into the mix. However, one thing for sure is that experiencing too much stress for too long is detrimental to our brain, body, health and how we feel, and can create a big dip on your metaphorical rollercoaster ride.

Chronic stress can throw your body budget into severe deficit. Your brain and body ramp up and continue overpredicting threat, activating your sympathetic nervous system even when not required. While short-term cortisol release can boost immunity and have a positive effect, over a long period it impacts on nearly every body system and is associated with poorer health and mood. All this can leave you feeling exhausted, burnt out and bad long term, with body budget deposits making little difference because you are so far into the red.

Human to human, our bodies and brains are all interlinked, which means you have a powerful impact on those around you, and vice versa. Constant criticism from others makes frequent withdrawals from our body budget and means we are more likely to predict this in the future. Your manager's words in a meeting can create calm or threat, and affect your body, depending on what they say and do (and have done in the past). A partner returning home might calm you down or increase your threat response, depending on your relationship and therefore what your brain is predicting.

While feeling unsafe can create deficits in your body budget, feeling safe can help create deposits. Your context is an important part of feeling safe, but perhaps most important are your connections – the people riding alongside you on your emotional rollercoaster. Having safe social relationships creates deposits, which helps regulate the body and reduce the negative impact of stress. We are social creatures, we perceive other people's emotions and they can also create emotions in us, as our bodies and brains respond to them and their emotions. There are many examples of this. Sitting quietly with someone can help slow their heartbeat; holding hands can make you feel safe; cuddling a crying child helps calm them down. The words we use also create body sensations: saying 'I love you' impacts on our physiology. Through our actions and words, we can co-regulate and help manage our body budget.

The following exercises are designed to help you manage the emotions arising from stress and learn how to use co-regulation and connection to influence your emotions.

Signs of stress

Stressors are inevitable and not always bad, yet too many or long-term stress can be harmful. It's important to notice your signs of stress as they can be an indicator that something needs to be tackled or thought about. Use the following examples and the image below to consider and then write out a list of your signs of stress, so you can start to learn to think about your needs.

Possible physical signs: tense muscles, fatigue, headaches.

Possible behaviour signs: changes in sleep or appetite, increased snappiness or irritability.

Possible thinking and feeling signs: difficulty concentrating, racing thoughts, feeling overwhelmed, difficulty making decisions, feeling anxious or worried

physical signs

thinking + feeling signs

behaviour signs

SIGNS YOUR STRESS FLAG IS FLYING

It's heavy

Stressor flags

How you respond to stressors can help reduce or increase them. We all want to run away from difficult feelings at times, but research shows that consistent avoidance is bad for our wellbeing. However, your emotions and your mood will improve if you identify your stressors and find helpful ways to respond. Use the illustration on page 56 to identify the situations which you know create a stress response in you and then think which of the ideas might work in response.

Co-regulation

This is a powerful tool to help regulate how we feel, put deposits into our body budget and support difficult emotions. Use these prompts to think about how you can use co-regulation effectively for your emotions.

• *Who comforts me when I feel stressed or overwhelmed?* Think about this in different situations, such as work or home.

• *Do certain people help co-regulate me in particular situations or times of day?* (e.g. cuddling your children after a stressful day at work)

• *What do they do that helps comfort me?* This might be talking through your feelings, a simple action such as a hug, or even just being in their presence.

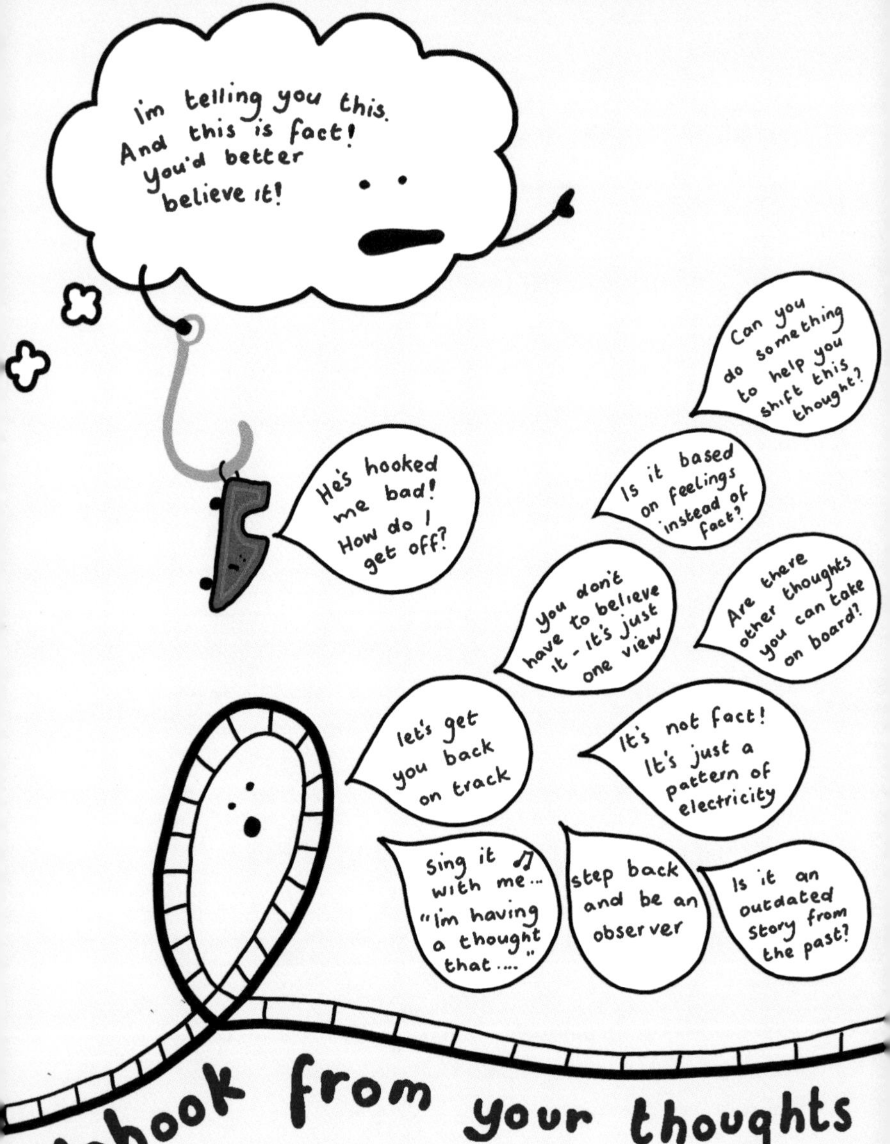
I'm telling you this. And this is fact! You'd better believe it!
He's hooked me bad! How do I get off?
Can you do something to help you to shift this thought?
Is it based on feelings instead of fact?
You don't have to believe it - it's just one view
Are there other thoughts you can take on board?
let's get you back on track
It's not fact! It's just a pattern of electricity
Sing it ♫ with me… "I'm having a thought that…."
step back and be an observer
Is it an outdated story from the past?
Unhook from your thoughts

The thinking brain

Thoughts are strange things, constantly passing through our mind every waking minute. Even when you think you are doing nothing, your brain is hard at work thinking over what's been, what will be and what might be. Our thoughts travel to the past and the future and even create imaginary worlds that have never and can never exist. Thoughts might be in the form of images or words or both. Sometimes thoughts shout at us, but they also frequently seem ephemeral and hard to capture. So, if we get down to basics, what are thoughts?

Remember those millions of neurons with their trillions of connections (see page 50)? At their most basic, thoughts are electrical impulses linking neurons to fire together in patterns. They are constructed by linking representations in your brain, providing you with constructs and understanding of sensory information. Your thoughts could be viewed as a window between your mind and the world, capturing some of the incoming data, filtered by the focus of your attention and framed by your experience, predictions and the constructs that exist in your mind. Thoughts are not static: they move and fluctuate. We can change and influence them, creating new links, learning which window to keep looking through and recognizing which are unhelpful to us – due to the beliefs, mood and experiences which frame them. We can decide to widen or transform some of these windows; or we can choose to look through another window entirely.

Estimates of how many thoughts we have a day vary from a few thousand to a hundred thousand. A 2020 study stated that we have about 6,200 'thought worms' per day. Yes that's right, thought worms – the moments when your brain activity (the content of your thoughts) would noticeably change under a brain scanner. However many we have, they are constant companions on our rollercoaster, linked intrinsically with our emotions. In fact, it is our very thoughts that define an instance of emotion, by categorizing all the data coming at your brain and conceptualizing this through our language. Traditional views may say that thoughts trigger emotions, but in reality it's a two-way ride. Sometimes our thoughts push the rollercoaster along a particular path, with feelings and resulting instances of emotions arising from thoughts. Other times, our emotions power the rollercoaster, driving our thoughts, transforming these according to how we feel. This is no surprise: both thoughts and emotions are products of information processing, so they go hand-in-hand along the rollercoaster, one sometimes exerting more pull on the other, and working together to understand your world.

How we feel, and our associated emotions, play a key biological role in our information processing, which influences thoughts. Let's look at how this happens. We know by now that our brain and body functioning are intertwined with how we feel. Anyone who has ever felt physically anxious will have noticed the effects on their thinking – being on high alert or unable to think clearly. Research shows when we feel anxious, we are more likely to predict a negative outcome to seemingly ambiguous information. This makes sense. If you live in a threatening environment, you need to become attuned to threat quickly. When we feel good, we are more likely to broaden our perspective, form social connections and decide to take chances, and our thoughts will align with this. When we feel sad, our executive functioning (the manager of your brain that does planning, problem-solving, etc.) is impacted, and this includes attention, which can impact on memory. Our thinking also becomes consistent with our mood – we notice the negative more, and have difficulty making decisions or coming up with solutions. Think about a time when you or someone you know has been depressed. You may notice self-criticism increases, getting stuck on a topic is common, and solutions or ideas may reduce. When our emotions are on a downward dip, our thoughts go with them.

Our thinking can influence our body, how we feel – and can create emotions, too. Our predictions may come out in our thoughts ('I'm not going to that social event, it will be terrible, no one will want to speak to me') and this influences how our body responds, in tension and rigidity. What goes on in our mind creates physical sensation – our brain doesn't differentiate between whether the data is external or internal to us. If you criticize yourself frequently, this is akin to having a bully walking alongside you. Blaming yourself for every bad thing that happens, or thinking you are doomed to fail, can make you feel doomed inside. If you imagine yourself in a happy place (as sometimes suggested in yoga or meditation, for example) then your body will respond to that vision, in your thoughts. You will slow down, you will feel calm. When it comes to emotions and thinking, it is a seesaw cycle of physiology affecting thinking, and thinking affecting physiology, all creating sensations and data that feed into our personal recipe of emotions.

How our brain has learned to respond comes from our upbringing and experience, and we might be predisposed to think in certain ways in certain situations. Sometimes a memory seems to pop up out of nowhere – and boom, we get the associated emotions. Great, if it is the holiday of your dreams, not so great if it is memory of trauma or sadness. Sometimes we start predicting threat before we've even realized we're doing it: 'I'm going to mess up this presentation.' While we can't always predict what thoughts will arise on our emotional rollercoaster, we *can* have more agency in how we respond. We can also find ways to redirect our thinking; in other words, make the rollercoaster take a slightly different route to create a different set of responses.

What's my thought worm telling me?

I like the idea of thought worms, travelling around our brain. The ones that capture your attention will differ, as some emerge into your awareness, and others fade into the soil. There may be many at once; or some might keep reappearing, no matter how much you'd rather they vanished. Although our thoughts can be unpleasant at times, pushing them away has the effect of making them pop up more, like a beachball that you try to push under the water. Seeing them helps our thoughts be heard and understood, and recognized for what they are – stories that we can choose to engage with, or not – rather than letting them dictate. By acknowledging them, we are able to influence how we interact with them, how we feel about them and how they make us feel.

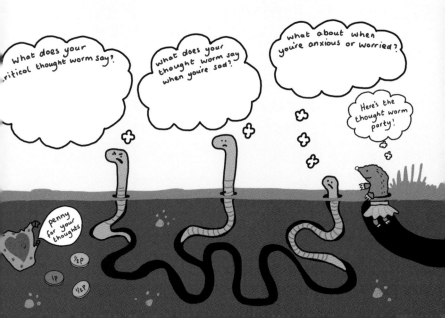

How will we frame it?

You are not your thoughts, and your thoughts are not fact. If a thought is troubling you, then frame it. This is your current frame on the world, but there are many others through which you can look that can help to shift your viewpoint. Reframing your perspective is beneficial for wellbeing. Use the prompts in the image opposite to frame your troubling thought and think how your situation might alter if you adjust your viewpoint to one of the other frames. Notice how this shift makes you feel.

Unhooking from your thoughts

Some thoughts can be hard to shake off. We get entangled in them and they become an intrinsic part of the rollercoaster ride. Sometimes we might not have the energy to interrogate our thoughts. We might have used other techniques already, or recognize they are unhelpful thoughts emerging because we are feeling down. Sometimes we just need a break from them. If thoughts are making you feel rubbish, you may need to encourage your brain to engage in something else for a while. This isn't about avoidance; it's about choosing to shift your focus. You can do this through activities that engage you and provide pleasure. Use the image on page 64 to think about ways to unhook from your thoughts, and give your brain a break, shifting your cognitive resources to somewhere more helpful for you.

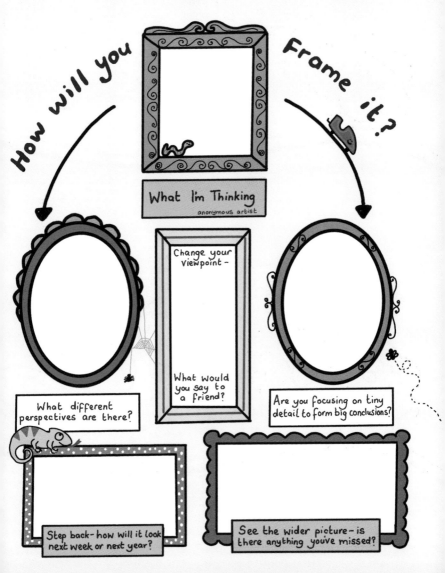

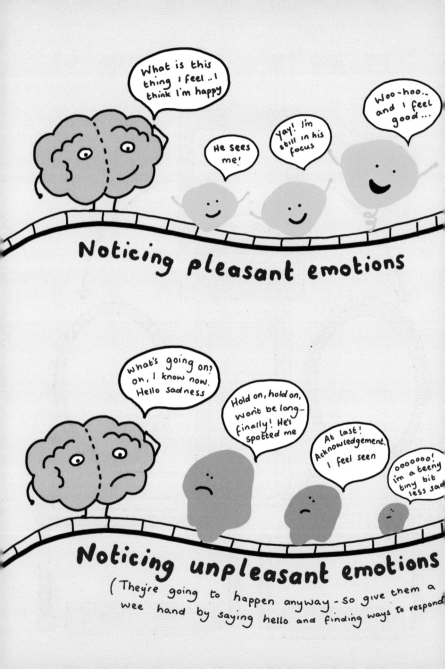

Chapter 3

Responding to Our Emotions

Hold on tight! Your emotional rollercoaster is heading towards a steep downhill trajectory – what do you do now? We might not always be able to decide where it takes us – as we've seen in the last chapters, many factors outside our control feed into how we feel. However, we do have more agency in how we respond when our rollercoaster takes us on an unpleasant dive or loop-the-loop. Our responses to our emotions can either help us navigate that route and come out the other end or get us stuck on a looped bit of track, unable to move forward. However, we first need to spot our emotions, and that's not always as easy as you might think. All too often we try to pretend our rollercoaster is on a smooth ride through life, suppressing, denying and ignoring any deviations on its course, which means we don't always know what we are feeling or why. This can feel like a good technique to keep our rollercoaster running smoothly, but ultimately it tends to fight back with unexpected bumps, stalling or outbursts on the ride. This chapter looks at how we can spot our emotions as we ride along the tracks and how our responses can help the rollercoaster run more smoothly.

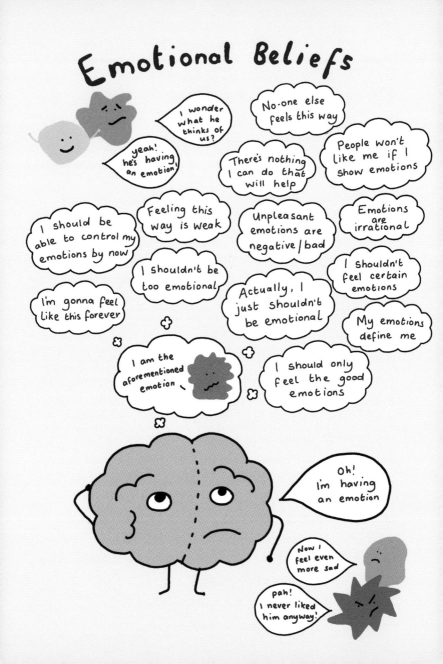

Our learned response
to emotions

We've thought about thoughts and how they drive your emotional rollercoaster, but there's an important type of thought that is central to your rollercoaster journey: your beliefs about emotions themselves. This really does affect how we experience them and what we do when they arise. Have you ever told yourself to 'pull yourself together' or that you have 'no right' to feel this way? Or perhaps you tell yourself that you 'should be happy' given all the good things in your life? As you head down into a dip, do you admonish yourself for not coping? Or as your anger rises, do you tell yourself that anger is unhelpful and to just calm the heck down? These are your beliefs about emotions creeping through your thoughts, affecting how you interact with the highs and lows of your rollercoaster, how you respond to your emotions and what you do when the ride deviates from a straight line (because it will). These beliefs are so powerful they can in fact steer our rollercoaster and create emotions all by themselves. Our beliefs can even get us stuck in a loop, prolong our downs (or ups) and produce secondary emotions in response to the initial emotions we experience.

Our beliefs develop through the messages we receive from family, friends, colleagues, magazines, television and culture, etc. The stories we hear, see and experience become *our* stories, which influence what we think and do. Understanding our beliefs about emotions is crucial, if we want to help shift where our rollercoaster takes us in the future.

We've already looked at stories you have heard and societal myths that exist around emotions, and these are likely to have fed into your beliefs. Think about them now (see Exercise 1 on page 79 to help with this): what are the messages you have previously received about emotions and how do these link to what you believe now? Was it only acceptable to show so-called positive emotions? Were emotions dismissed? Were you given messages about particular emotions? For example, that anger is unacceptable and pride or jealousy make you a bad person? Were certain emotions only acceptable in some people? For example, were women criticized for being too emotional or was anger acceptable only in men? Was crying something to be ashamed of? Were you considered bad if you were anxious or angry? Or were difficult emotions something you needed to push aside and try to fix? We have all received messages about emotions both directly (such as punishing them or being told it's okay to feel emotions) or covertly (such as ignoring them, distracting from emotions or needing to fix them as soon as possible).

These messages shape our beliefs. How your emotions were responded to early in life will influence how you respond to them now, which is why it is crucial to help children understand their emotions. The stories of what emotions are and how you should respond to them will be influenced by the time, place and culture in which you have lived.

Of course, these beliefs shape how we experience, understand and respond to our emotions, and how we show our emotions (or not) – our 'display rules'. These are the implicit or explicit rules for showing our emotions, which form our general pattern of responding to emotions. Have we learned to bottle them up (such as hiding our tears while watching a sad movie), or do we only ever discuss positive emotions? As we'll see in the next topic, some of these display rules that we have learned to follow may be unhelpful and, ironically, create even more difficult emotions.

All of these deep-rooted beliefs and rules come out in our thinking when we experience an emotion. What you think and believe about your own emotions can influence the next emotion you feel. These are sometimes called 'secondary emotions': those that occur because of how we respond to our initial emotions. They can sometimes be extremely unhelpful, creating spirals on your rollercoaster that lead you further down into a black hole. If you berate or criticize yourself for experiencing emotions, you are not going to make yourself feel good. Your brain will most likely feel threatened or despondent, and that will play out in your emotions, which amplifies any difficult feelings you already had. Similarly, shaming yourself for having an emotion (for example, berating yourself for being 'too' upset over a passing criticism) will not make you feel good, and will lead to more difficult feelings.

Beliefs about whether we can cope when emotions arise are important, too, for how we respond. If you believe emotions are out of your control, you are more likely to feel anxious and less likely to respond helpfully to them or use coping strategies that may make things better. But, if you feel like you have some strategies to help you deal with your emotions and know what to do when they arise, they feel less scary. People who see emotions as something they can tackle feel more in control, which impacts positively on how they feel, thereby reducing the power of challenging emotions when they do arrive.

The stories we tell ourselves about our own emotions are often behind the driving wheel of our responses and can either allow us to navigate through these emotions helpfully or drive us onto a negative loop of track. We can learn to update our stories about emotions so our beliefs become more helpful to us. The following exercises are designed to help you identify your beliefs about emotions and challenge them to help you drive your emotional rollercoaster in a more supportive direction.

I'm an emotional believer

Many of the beliefs we hold about emotions come from our upbringing, as well as the wider society and culture to which we belong. Use the image on page 74 to help you think about the messages you may have received about emotions up to this point. These can be direct, from what people have told you or indirect, from the way in which those around you have reacted to emotions. Now, think about how these messages have shaped your beliefs. Note down some of the thoughts – and judgements – that come to mind when you think about emotions. What do you say to yourself (or others) when experiencing different emotions, and what do you do in response? These are great clues to identify your beliefs about the emotions themselves. If you are having difficulty (beliefs can be notoriously hard to spot), I've included a few in the image on page 74 that I often hear in my work as a psychologist. See if you recognize any of these in yourself.

Your display rules

Use the following prompts to think about how those messages and your beliefs about emotions have impacted on your display rules.

• Make a list of common emotions and describe what your outward display would look like? Do you have general display rules, or are they specific to different emotions (e.g. 'I can display happiness, but not too much' or 'I should never show pride')?

• What messages did you receive as you grew up (or currently) about how emotions should or shouldn't be shown (e.g. 'Anger is unacceptable')?

• What do your display rules tell you about how you should respond to or show emotions? Were you surprised at the results? Are there some emotions that take a lot of effort to suppress? If so, what would be a reasonable release?

Debunking your emotional myths

Just as bad science needs to be debunked, our emotional beliefs based on unhelpful beliefs also need to be debunked. Let's use this scientific experiment opposite to come up with some new beliefs about emotions, which you can apply in your own life.

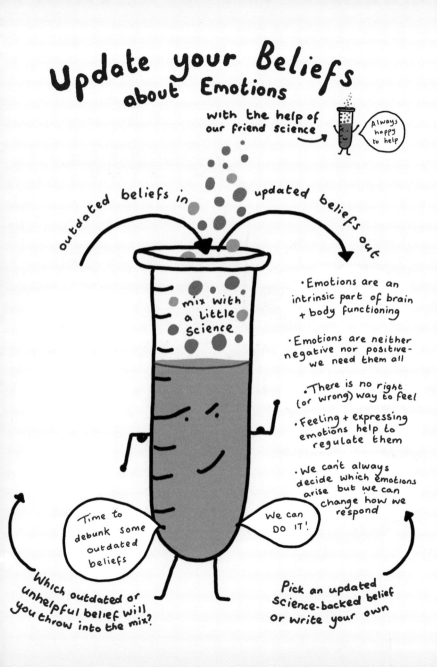

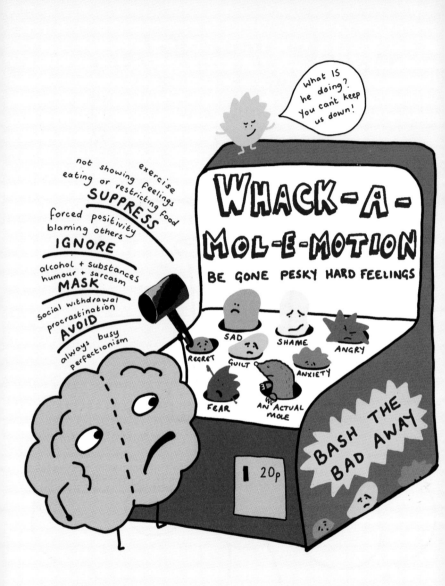

Just go away

Life is tough at times, and it's inevitable that your emotional rollercoaster will experience some nose-dives through difficult periods and emotions. No one gets through life without feeling tough or unpleasant emotions at some point. But unlike on a real-life rollercoaster, no one raises their hands and cheers as they roll into these feel-bad stretches of track. It's an interesting fact that we have far more words for so-called negative emotions than positive emotions. These emotions fall into the left-hand side of the emotional compass (see page 90), as they all describe unpleasant feelings. Yet, despite having far more words for them, we tend to speak about them less. Often, we don't want to focus on them at all and find ways to push them away or avoid them. It's the most natural thing in the world to try to get away from something unpleasant. Unfortunately, it's not so easy to shut away the feelings that exist in our brain and body. In fact, this tends to make them come back stronger, or pop out in ways we don't expect.

One of the main reasons we want to get away from crappy emotions is obvious – no one wants to feel rubbish. I've never met anybody who said, 'It was great when I felt really anxious the other day' or 'I had a wonderful time when I was depressed'. We may also feel ill-equipped to deal with them; they might make us feel out of control; or we might feel fearful that if we let them in, we will make them worse. Alternatively, we might think we just don't have time to deal with these pesky difficult emotions that disrupt our busy life. Our beliefs play a role too: we may think we *shouldn't* be feeling this way so push it aside, or we might try to mask our feelings because we believe that feeling good is the only acceptable emotion to display. Let's be honest, we are never going to open our arms and welcome our difficult emotions, but we don't need to push them away either. Instead of battling with them, we can learn to sit alongside them, with acceptance that they are an inevitable and necessary part of life. Research shows this can help stop the dips lurching down further.

The ironic thing about suppressing emotions is that it has the opposite effect to what we hope to achieve. Research shows it doesn't actually make us feel better at all, but rather amplifies our difficult emotions. If I asked you to avoid thinking about a bar of chocolate you have in the cupboard (or for me, crisps), I bet the more you try not to think about it, the more it pops into your mind at every random occasion (I'm certainly thinking of crisps now). Psychological experiments demonstrate that trying hard *not* to focus on something brings it to our attention far more (I'm still thinking of the crisps). It also uses a heap of cognitive resources and energy, so can place a lot of demand on the brain. Suppressing emotions or thoughts increases our physiological stress response, and, conversely, expressing them reduces stress. It's not that we never need to avoid emotions – sometimes distraction is just what we need – but if this becomes our normal response, it can become unhelpful, and is associated with poor wellbeing.

Avoiding our emotions can come in many forms. We might deny their existence and refuse to notice how we are feeling, or we might busy ourselves doing other things so we don't have to feel them. We might know they are there but push them down, never showing them or talking about them – trying not to let them sneak out at any cost. Or we might get into a battle with them: telling them we shouldn't be feeling like this and we just need to pull ourselves together. The Harvard psychologist Dr Susan David describes this avoidance or suppression as 'bottling', where you hold your emotions at arm's length, which is exhausting physically, making them feel heavy and likely to drop unexpectedly. Unfortunately, these emotions often pop out anyway. You might end up shouting at your kids when actually your frustration lies somewhere else, or snap at a colleague when the issue is being undermined by somebody else in the meeting you've just attended.

Alternatively, perhaps the opposite happens and your emotions stick to you, and you get overwhelmed by them. Susan David describes this as 'brooding' – another unhelpful way we respond to emotions – which is when we hold our emotions so tightly, like a book to the chest, and are so caught up in them, we can never separate ourselves from them. Again, brooding is associated with poorer wellbeing and more difficulty negotiating the challenging stuff that life throws at our emotional rollercoaster ride. Different areas of psychology use different terminology for getting stuck in your emotions – you could also think of it as getting *hooked* by or *stuck* in the emotion (see The Thinking Brain, page 64), so we have difficulty moving through it or learning from it. It's our rollercoaster stalling because of debris on the track.

This debris can take a number of forms. Perhaps we get stuck in the thoughts that come with our emotions, ruminating perpetually on our uncertain future; or we've just got so much stressful stuff on the tracks that we are stuck in overwhelm – frozen and unable to move forward. The cognitive effect of feeling bad can itself keep us stuck: difficulty with decision-making may mean we can see no solutions; difficulty with flexible thinking may mean we struggle to shift to another perspective; and difficulty with attention may mean we don't notice the stuff that could help us feel good. Or it might be that we don't recognize the emotion we are experiencing, so struggle to stand back and observe how it's impacting on us. These blockages on the tracks can keep us stuck in the emotion, unable to step out of it onto another path or move through it.

There is a middle ground between these two extreme responses that helps us step back, recognize our emotions and hold them lightly, rather than being driven by them. We'll look at this in the next few topics. However, in order to get there, we need to assess and understand how we currently respond to those emotions that make us feel negative. Let's look at your responses to emotions.

Do you bottle or brood?

We all have different emotional responses at different times, but we may notice patterns that characterize our responses. These are not mutually exclusive – you may notice that you tend to get hooked on emotions that arise in certain situations or with particular people but studiously avoid others. Use the image opposite to think about your response patterns. If you have noticed you get stuck in emotions, recognizing factors that contribute to this is the first step to shifting some of the debris from the track.

Avoidance by many forms

Avoidance is when we try to not experience an emotion by distracting ourselves. Think about ways that you avoid emotions. Some distractions can be helpful, but like all coping strategies it can depend on their function. Does this distraction help to support you with difficult emotions and help you respond to them, or is it used to simply block them out? Exercise is a great example of this – it has a good evidence base for helping improve depression and reduce anxiety, and often people feel it helps clear their mind. Yet, I have worked with people who use exercise excessively to block out all those bad emotions, in which case it may be unhelpful. Look over the items listed on the image on page 82 and consider whether you use them to block out emotions or to support your emotions (of course, this may vary on different occasions).

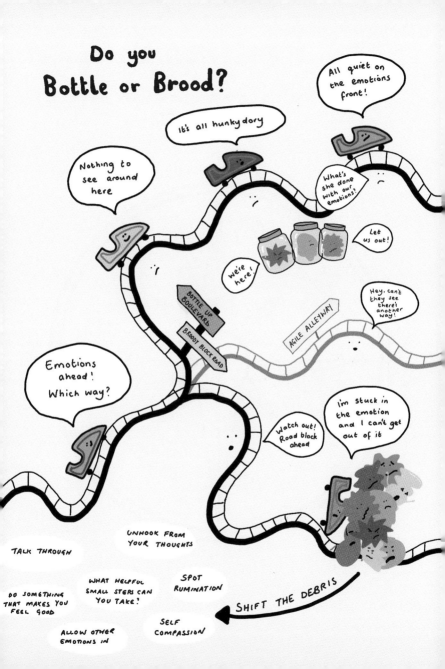

The Feelings Compass

Which direction is your affect?

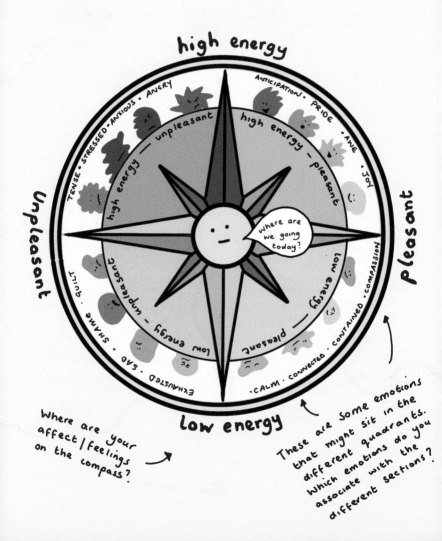

Where are your affect/feelings on the compass?

These are some emotions that might sit in the different quadrants. Which emotions do you associate with the different sections?

Spot your emotions

I remember a competition in our Saturday newspaper when I was little called Spot the Ball. It was a photo of a football match with the ball removed, and you won the competition by guessing correctly where the ball was. Sounds easy, but there were lots of decoys – the players were usually looking in the wrong direction and the ball was never where you thought it would be. I diligently completed it every week but was never successful. I think spotting your emotions is a bit like Spot the Ball – it sounds easy but is often deceptively hard. Luckily, I've become a bit more successful at spotting my emotions over the years.

As we've seen through our emotional cookies (see page 32), how we feel in our body is at the core of emotions. The body constantly feeds data to us, and we understand this through a process of interoception. We may get specific feedback, such as a sore stomach or pain in our head, or we may experience a summary of what's going on via our affect, which is our brain judging the overall state of our body budget. We build on this to understand what's going on, be that emotional or physical need, and what to do about it. However, it's not as easy as it sounds. Think back to your emotional beliefs – many of us have been taught by the culture we grew up in not to listen to our body. When we fall, we've been told to 'be a big boy' or to 'just get up and dust yourself off'. Our attention may also have been drawn to our cognitive world (our thoughts) and our external world, so we never notice what's going on in our body.

Many of us have learned to ignore the internal signals our body is giving us, because the demands of the external world feel too great. Sometimes this becomes so bad that we ignore even the urge to pee, or a rumbling stomach indicating hunger. I know from working in a busy hospital that it's all too common to be caught up in your day and ignore signs of thirst to the point you are so dehydrated it impacts negatively on your mood. You tell yourself that your body just needs to hold on while you get on with the important business of being a busy human. However, it is crucial to notice and understand the demands of your body. Not only are these at the root of emotions, providing essential information to indicate how you feel, but also, at the most basic level, responding to your body's (very reasonable) demands is the foundation for self-care. Feeding our body when it tells us to, peeing when we need to, resting when required and letting our body recover when unwell are all key to keeping a healthy body budget, making us feel good and stay well.

As well as ignoring our body sensations, we can also learn to mask them. I like a daily coffee, but I only started drinking it when my children were little, due to severe sleep deprivation: when it gave me a much-needed boost to get through the day. A few years on it had become a habit, every time I passed the hospital coffee shop, they had my latte at the ready. I'm not sure if I recognized how tired I was, as it was masked by my too-regular coffees, meaning I just kept on going and not resting when my body told me I needed to. It's this shift from a helpful short-term boost to a repeated masking of how we feel that starts to impact negatively on how we manage our body budget. We can mask how we feel in many ways, with drugs, alcohol, pain relief, over-exercising, and food being the most common.

It sounds cheesy to say 'listen to your body', but it's giving you important data. That data might be showing you need to manage your body budget in some way (with relaxation, sleep, going for a pee, eating something, or drinking more water). Yet, as our mind and body are intrinsically intertwined, we can't really separate the sensations of hunger or thirst from what we would describe as emotions. The feelings resulting from these body sensations can make us feel rubbish, which we might label as sad, frustrated or anxious. Looking after your emotions can sometimes feel intangible, but noticing your body signs and responding to your physical needs is a huge part of it. This is not a new idea – traditional yoga practices focus on bringing your attention to the body to notice and understand what's going on. However, our modern world tends to override our focus on our body, as we shift into our busy minds to deal with the hectic pace of life. Many Western therapies often encourage us to look at how our mind impacts on us, with less consideration of the equally important physical aspects of emotions.

As well as helping you manage your body budget, listening to your body provides a whole host of other data that helps you understand yourself, your world and how you can respond to it. It helps us identify when we are overloaded with stress, or when something is difficult in life and we need to take care of ourselves. It guides us towards what is meaningful, what engages us, what calms us. Ignoring these signs can lead to overwhelm and poor health, and suppressing or shaming emotions amplifies them. Getting to know them helps us live with and learn from our emotions and respond to them helpfully. We can stand back from them, observe them and guide them, rather than feeling they drive us.

Once we notice what's going on in our body, we need to make sense of it. What do butterflies in your stomach mean? What does the ache in your shoulders signify? Why are you feeling 'bleurgh' this morning? How we attribute meaning is important. Research shows that our interpretations are not always accurate. We can mistake a churning stomach from illness for feeling excited or attracted to someone. We are only ever taking a best guess at what these feelings mean, but noticing them regularly helps us understand them better.

A quick word of caution: while getting to understand how you feel in your body is essential to your emotions, there may be times when you are so acutely aware of your interoceptive senses that this feels unhelpful. For example, when suffering with social anxiety, we are very focused on how we feel internally and whether others observe this; or with health anxiety, we are acutely aware of any indications of poor health or panic attacks, and observations of our body can feed into sensations of panic. If you find your internal focus is unhelpful or oppressive for you, it may be that getting to understand your body better may need to be done in a supportive therapeutic space.

The feelings compass

Let's start by getting to know your brain's summary of your body budget (affect or mood) using the feelings compass on page 90. This can help you notice how you are feeling and start to make sense of it. Use the compass when you notice something's going on, or at regular points throughout the day to get to know your mood better. We don't conceptualize all feelings as emotions, so this may help you identify other factors contributing to how you are feeling, too. For example, if you are constantly feeling tired, do you need to get a health check or focus on your sleep?

Listen to your body's data

Beyond that general sense of how we are doing, we may also get more specific data from our body, such as the physical signs of stress. Listening to this data helps manage your body budget as well as understand your emotions. Use the image opposite to identify where you are experiencing sensations in your body and use the word cloud to help describe them. Ask yourself how you are feeling a few times a day, so you can begin to listen to what your body is telling you (try using the mental body scan method from Exercise 1 on page 54 to help with this). Once you notice what's going on in your body, consider what it is telling you to do. Is it saying, 'Hey, I need a snack, a pee, a rest, or a few deep breaths'? Take action to help keep your body budget in balance.

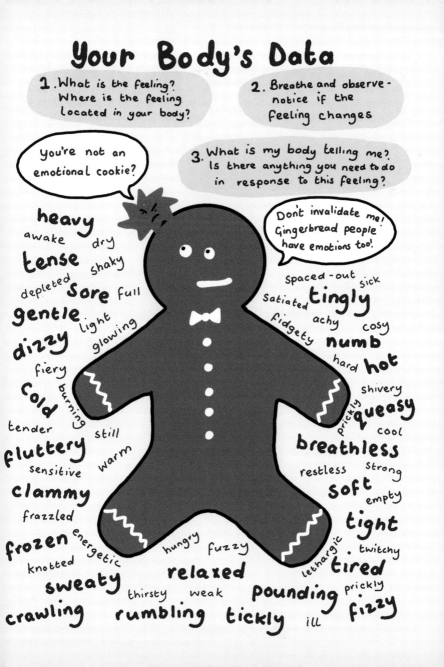

Sieve your Emotions

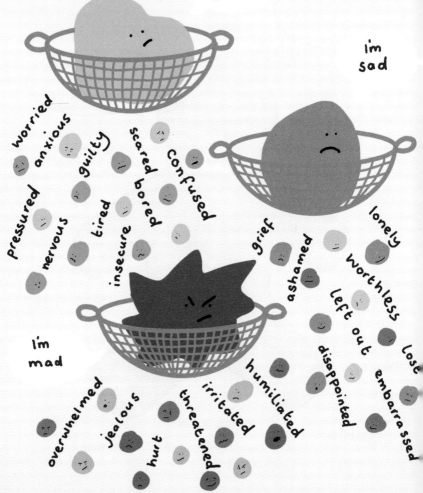

Express yourself

I've always been intrigued by the way snow is described in different languages, and my children are tickled by the so-called fact that the Inuits have fifty words for snow. Although this may not be true (linguists can argue about this), the way we understand the concept of snow differs around the world. Just like snow, some emotion words only exist in certain languages. A commonly known one is *schadenfreude* – joy or satisfaction from someone else's misfortune. Most of us will recognize this, but without this wonderful German word we might be unable to put a name to it or conceptualize it. Cultures categorize and conceptualize our emotional world differently, and different languages recognize different emotions. Our concepts are crucial for emotions, as they affect not only what we are able to communicate, but also how we internally perceive, understand and respond to our emotional world.

Emotions are the concepts we use to give our internal sensations meaning. The words and definitions that exist in our language shift this endless stream of data into categories so we can understand and construct meaning from it. Constructs don't just apply to emotions, of course; they apply to our whole world and existence. Our brain is always using its pre-existing concepts in the form of words to match the data coming our way with past experiences, to make sense of them. We see and make sense of the world with these concepts, and they provide structure, but they're not static – we are constantly building on our verbal constructs to help us understand new information. Very few people before 2020 would have understood 'social distancing', for example, yet we learned new concepts to help us deal with and understand this new information. Each time we start a new job or go to a new country, we will learn new concepts to define and understand the new information we come across, and we encode this into our memory so we can define future data better. As you've seen through my collection of emotions, we can do this with emotions, too, and our brain (and body) will thank us for it.

I recently heard researcher Brené Brown on The Happiness Lab podcast (see Further Reading, page 188), quoting the philosopher Ludwig Wittgenstein, who wrote, 'The limits of my language mean the limits of my world.' Having a wider range of concepts in our vocabulary widens our world, meaning we can understand the world in a more nuanced way. This is particularly relevant for our emotional world, yet many of us have a limited emotional vocabulary. Describing her research with 70,000 people, Brown found that many could only name and recognize their experiences as three broad emotional terms: mad (i.e. angry), sad and glad (happy). Many of us tend to define our emotions with broad brushstrokes, such as 'I'm so angry', 'I feel great' or 'I'm so stressed out', rather than going into the nitty gritty. These non-specific terms can encompass a broad range of feelings and experiences. If we put these emotions through a sieve and divided them into their component parts, we'd most likely find that multiple experiences contribute to these feelings. This can help us understand our experience in more detail. For example, anger at one point in time (perhaps furious at an observed injustice) would look different from anger at another point (snapping at your child when your brain is overloaded).

Breaking your emotions down into detail is called 'emotional granularity', and some people construct finer-grained emotional experiences than others. Lisa Feldman-Barrett describes how people range from high emotional granularity (able to describe many emotional experiences) to low emotional granularity (only able to describe limited terms). Emotional granularity is not just about building a vocabulary, however, it's also about being able to apply these words to your experiences to help understand them better and know what to do about them. Our rollercoaster can get stuck when we don't have the language or constructs to describe our experiences. It can make us less likely to communicate, conceptualize and share our experiences. Longer term, lower granularity may be linked to those downward spirals on our rollercoaster, as it's associated with increased depression, anxiety and other mental health concerns. It can mean that difficult life events have a greater negative impact, and that we have more difficulty regulating emotions and fewer coping strategies in response to emotions.

Emotional granularity is a key mechanism in understanding our emotions. Having increased granularity means you can predict better; spot, understand and regulate emotions; and be able to put in place the helpful responses that support your rollercoaster. Increasing granularity gives your brain the gift of being able to make better sense of those sensations that pop up every day, so it can be more flexible in how it responds to them. This has positives for not just how you respond to emotions, but how you feel generally – naming an emotion appears to reduce stress. It helps manage your body budget, as better predictions require less cognitive effort to respond to your needs. And we know that a well-maintained and balanced body budget impacts positively on how we feel and our health. Not only do people with high granularity appear to be able to regulate their emotions better and are more likely to use helpful coping strategies, they also appear to have better health (because of the body budget implications) and get ill less frequently (because physical health is intrinsically tied to how we feel). The benefits don't stop there. Higher granularity also appears to be linked to improved social relationships and, as we know connections are hugely important for how we feel on our rollercoaster, this can have positive knock-on effects.

Hopefully I've persuaded you that it's worth joining my emotions collector club. Increasing your vocabulary is a great start to increasing emotional granularity; understanding how emotions are categorized in other languages is not only fascinating, but also adds more concepts and categories that help us predict and understand our emotions better. But, a collection gathering dust is no use – we need to ensure we apply it to ourselves, by using our concepts to understand our experiences. I would argue the limits of your emotional words are the limits of your imagination, because creating your own concepts to describe your emotional world is just as helpful. I am well known for my 'NFMs' (no food moods), which is my description for the grumpiness and intolerance I feel when I haven't eaten. This is extremely helpful as friends and family will tell me, 'Oh, I think you are at risk of an NFM', prompting me to eat and feel better. I've also coined the term 'netflixless' for that emptiness and loss I feel when the last episode of a favourite box set finishes. Making up your own words can help categorize your experiences (and can be a fun game to play with your kids and set them up with an emotional vocabulary that will support them as they develop).

The following exercises are designed to help you think about how to finely grain your emotions and build up your emotional vocabulary, in order to help your rollercoaster progress smoothly along its journey and respond helpfully to those bumps on the track.

Sieve your emotions

Next time you find yourself using one of the big three (angry, sad or happy) or the catch-all term 'stressed', try to sieve through these words to see if you can describe the emotion more accurately. Use the image on page 98 to help you think about what you are actually feeling, and break this down into its component parts. Remember, when describing your emotions, you don't have to be confined to one word; we can often feel multiple, sometimes conflicting, emotions all at once. Picking and choosing a range of emotions can help capture the nuances of what you feel.

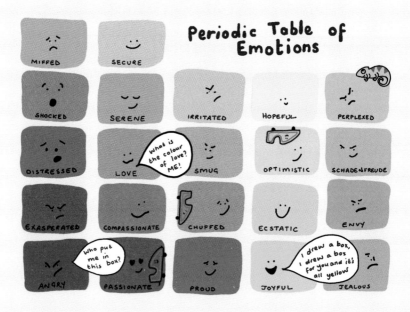

Become a collector of emotions

I started collecting emotions out of interest, little realizing that it would enable me to describe and understand my own emotions. There are some great tools to help you build up your emotional vocabulary; in the Further Reading section (see page 188) you'll find references to an emotional atlas and the feelings wheel. To persuade you to join my club, I've captured some of my collection in a Periodic Table of Emotions below. Use this as starter for your own collection and use your imagination for emotions that you have no name for. I would love to know what you come up with!

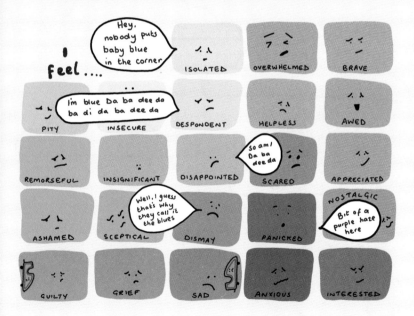

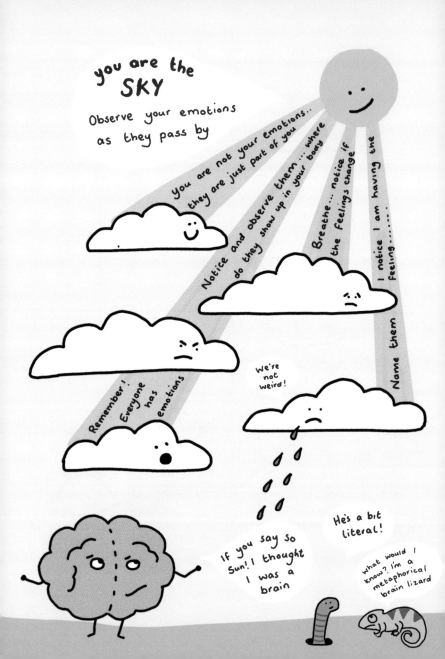

The space between emotion and action

Emotions are sources of information throughout life, telling us something about what's happening in the here and now, or why we are responding to the here and now in a particular way. I like psychologist Susan David's analogy of emotions as a lighthouse, providing data for how we need to navigate the world. Our emotional lighthouse is a natural guidance system, which provides signals that help us to navigate the choppy waters and avoid crashing onto the rocks. Data is coming at us throughout our life as our body and brain interact with the world around us and our brain predicts how it needs to respond. We've spent some time so far spotting this data and signals, as well as getting to know them better and shifting our beliefs about emotions to see them as a necessary and key component of our lives. While we can't always help which signals are emitted (the emotions that arise), we can have more control over how we respond. We've seen that ignoring the signals means our responses to our emotions are more likely to land us on the rocks, as it strengthens their force, meaning we can become driven by our emotions rather than understanding and thinking about how we respond to them. Learning instead to step back and create space from our emotions is a critical component so we can consider our next steps.

Before taking this step back though, we need to make friends with our emotions (or at least become empathetic acquaintances), and to do this we need to accept them for what they are. Our emotions will come into our world whether we want them to or not. Difficult emotions are stubborn little (or sometimes big) things, so they will usually do the opposite of what you tell them to do: telling them to go away makes them stronger; ignoring them means they will pop back unexpectedly. There's really only one way to help, and that's to accept them. Accepting rather than battling emotions creates a little distance from them, space that helps us navigate them. To do this, we need to apply our belief shifts (see page 81) to our own emotions, then acknowledge and accept them.

It can be helpful to view emotions simply as data that arises, neither good nor bad, just part of the pattern of life. Rather than something that makes us different or abnormal, we can recognize difficult emotions as part of common human experience. It's also helpful to recognize that emotions and associated thoughts are not facts; they are transient parts of your story that you can shift and respond to differently.

You can also detangle your sense of worth from your emotions. Emotions are not you: they are part of you, but they do not define you. I like Matt Haig's description of emotions as clouds, while you are the sky. This illustrates that emotions aren't static, they come and go. You are bigger than the clouds – they do not define you, they are merely part of you. Just like clouds, there are different shapes, but there are no wrong emotions, they are fundamentally a part of being human and having a body that is linked to a brain in an ever-changing and sometimes difficult world.

Acceptance of emotions forms a key part of many psychological therapies; if we start to understand our emotions, and see them as data rather than as an indicator of our worth, we can tolerate them better. Observing and allowing them, and understanding they will pass (and in fact are more likely to, if we *are* tolerant of them), makes emotions less scary, meaning we are less likely to push them away and more likely to connect with them and become curious about them.

Seeing yourself as the sky also starts to create distance from your thoughts and feelings, which is an important technique to help you unhook from your emotions (see page 70). Once we notice and accept our emotions, we can start to stand back and observe them, like those passing clouds. Creating space between us and the emotion gives us a chance to think about how we respond. This helps us tolerate the emotion, rather than being hooked in by it, and enables us to guide our responses. Noticing the emotion and naming it are the first steps to help us unhook.

It may seem simplistic, but the use of language can have a powerful impact on separating us from our thoughts and feelings. Rather than saying, 'I am angry', we can say, 'I am feeling angry' or 'I notice I am feeling angry'. By doing this, we immediately use our language to take a step back and recognize anger as a feeling, rather than being part of us. Similarly, with our thoughts, saying, 'I am an idiot' is much more powerful than 'I am having the thought that I am an idiot', or 'Look brain, I know I'm telling myself that old story that I'm an idiot again', or simply 'My brain is having the pattern of electrical pulses that emerges when I am feeling stressed or have made a mistake'. In addition, creating a story around the emotion can also help unhook from it. This can be by talking it through or writing it down – both have shown to help with emotional regulation. There are lots of techniques to create space that are used in different therapies, and I have included some more ideas in Exercise 2 on page 114.

Being curious and trying to make sense of our emotions are key parts of stepping back from them. Research indicates that applying curiosity to emotions helps us process and respond to them. Once we've spotted and named them, we can try to understand what's going on for us. What is your emotional cookie mix at that particular point, and what type of cookie is it creating? What is your brain predicting that's feeding into this? What is going on in your body? What are your thoughts telling you? What's the backstory? Is there anything in the past that has made you respond in this particular way, in this particular context, that has fed into your cookie?

Psychologists call this recipe a 'formulation'. There are many different types of formulation that exist, but all off them provide a structure to help you make sense of and understand your experience. My emotional cookie formulation isn't an official research-based formulation, but it's designed to work out what your brain is constructing at any point, and help you start to think about why. The more we do this, the more we are likely to start to see patterns in how we respond in particular situations, and this can help us predict differently and know what to do. However, it's important to note that our formulation of what is making us feel a particular way is only ever a best guess or hypothesis. The more we get to know our emotions, the better we are at these guesses, but sometimes, no matter how hard we try, we can't work out *why* we are feeling a bit 'bleurgh', and that's okay. We don't have to interrogate and intricately understand every single emotion we have. Sometimes, we just need to remember there are many reasons and physiological mechanisms behind why we might feel a bit yucky, and we're not aware of all these processes. No matter whether you can pinpoint a reason or not, tolerating, accepting and acknowledging these feelings, and thinking about how best to respond, is helpful.

Now we've created some space from our emotions, what next? Remember those books that Susan David spoke about (see page 85)? Sometimes we hold them too far away and they become heavy; sometimes we hold them so close they start to make our muscles ache. The in-between way is holding them lightly. David calls this emotional agility, being able to respond nimbly to our emotions. In different psychological therapies, this is given different names: acceptance and commitment therapy calls it flexibility; cognitive behaviour theory focuses on viewing your thoughts from different angles; while mindfulness encourages you to step back and become an observer of your thoughts.

While different therapies may apply different terminology, they have a common theme of encouraging you to step back and respond in a flexible way to your emotions and related thoughts. On our rollercoaster, this enables us to observe what is happening, consider it and decide how best to respond. Instead of getting stuck on one route that is no longer working for us, we can choose to diverge to a different path. We can roll *with* the emotion and then consider where we want to roll next, rather than letting it decide our track.

We've already covered many of the factors that help us be agile – noticing, naming, understanding, stepping back and considering our response. One way we can start to be agile is to look at what the emotional data is telling us about our needs. What is the lighthouse signalling that you need, and how can you best respond to this? Are you tired or stressed? Are the signals indicating that you need greater connection? Exercise 4 on page 116 includes questions you can ask when you notice your lighthouse emitting data, to help think about what it is signalling to you. Throughout the rest of the book we'll look at more strategies that support our ability to make our responses to emotions flexible, functional and fit for purpose. These strategies enable us to navigate tough times and appreciate, notice and even create scenic journeys towards good times.

Accept and connect

Accepting your emotions is about allowing and tolerating them rather than pushing them away. It's about giving yourself non-judgemental permission to feel, with the understanding that doing so helps you navigate your rollercoaster through them, channel them and use your emotions wisely, rather than letting them control you. Compassion towards your emotions helps you to connect to them and move forward. Here are some ideas of statements to help accept and connect with your emotions.

1. Notice it. Notice the emotion and name it. How is this emotion showing up for you at this moment?

2. Allow it. Breathe slowly and gently, and allow the emotion to just be. Observe what happens.

3. Accept it. Remind yourself that it is okay to have emotions – they are a normal part of brain and body functioning. They arise and pass as part of life.

Become the sky: create space

Once you've accepted and connected with your emotions, imagine you are the sky and your emotions are passing clouds. What might you say to become an observer, rather than being stuck on the clouds? How can you create space and step back? Use the ideas in the sunshine rays on page 106, but feel free to add your own.

The curious case of emotions

Being curious about your emotions can help you understand why they occur and what you can do about them. Use the illustration below to help you understand what emotions you are experiencing and what's contributing to the emotions mix. You can use this during an emotion or to reflect on how you've felt during the day.

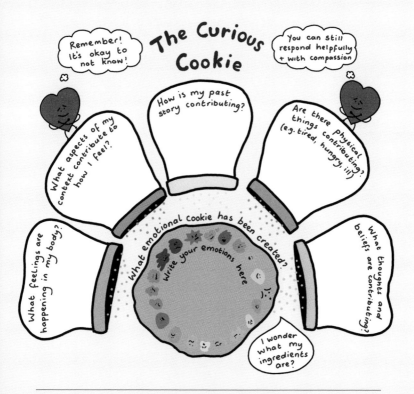

Emotions as signals

Ask yourself the questions in the lighthouse image to think about what your emotional data is signalling to you and how you might best respond. If we think of emotions as guiding signals this can point us to our needs and values. This exercise isn't just for tough emotions; the feel-good ones also give us information. We can use this to consider how we respond, both in the here and now and also more generally in our lives. For example, feeling distressed might indicate we need to do something immediately soothing, but may also mean that we need to do something about the cause of distress in the longer term. Perhaps someone has transgressed a boundary and we need to be clear about this in the future.

Here are some things that emotions might signal to you:
That we need more or less of something in our lives. For example, isolation may show we need greater connection, while overwhelm may indicate we need to evaluate our workplace demands.

That we are meeting our values or not meeting them; and we need to build on this. For example, feeling joy might show that we are doing something of value to us, while feeling hurt may indicate that someone is doing something that doesn't fit with our values.

That something needs to be tackled. Feeling stressed might be an indicator that we need support or that there are stressors we need to problem solve.

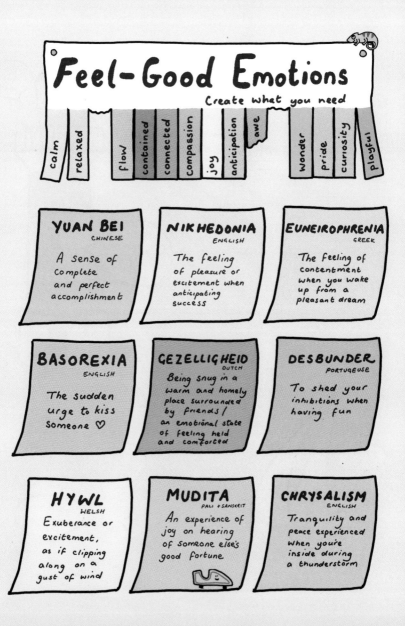

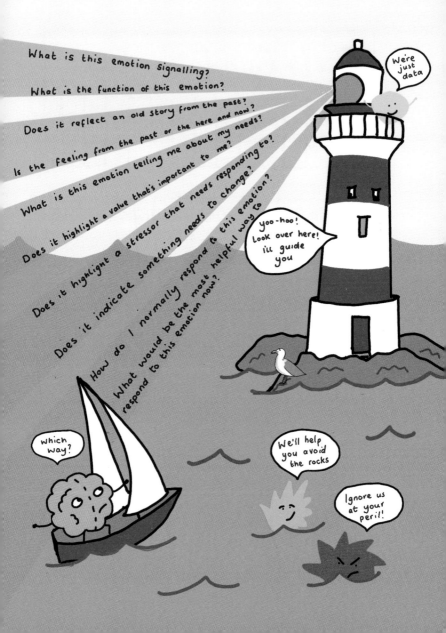

Chapter 4
Feel-Good Emotions

All emotions are required for life, and I try to steer away from categories of negative and positive emotions. However, we can create feelings and associated emotions that make us feel good – all those feelings that are on the right-hand side of the feelings compass (see page 90). There are a host of emotions we associate with feeling good, both upbeat and downbeat, and we know that experiencing these feel-good emotions is associated with improved wellbeing and health. There can be upbeat highs as our rollercoaster travels through awe-inducing landscapes, or gentle meandering paths through calming woods and waters, which bring peace of mind. However, your predicting threat-oriented brain tends to pull you towards the less pleasant feelings that arise on your rollercoaster. As a result, sometimes you may dash through the pleasant parts without even noticing them, or neglect or forget to drive to the places that make you feel good. Understanding emotions and what creates them means we can plan routes towards the ones we enjoy throughout our days, weeks and years. This chapter focuses on the emotions that make us feel good and how we can navigate, or signpost, our rollercoaster towards them.

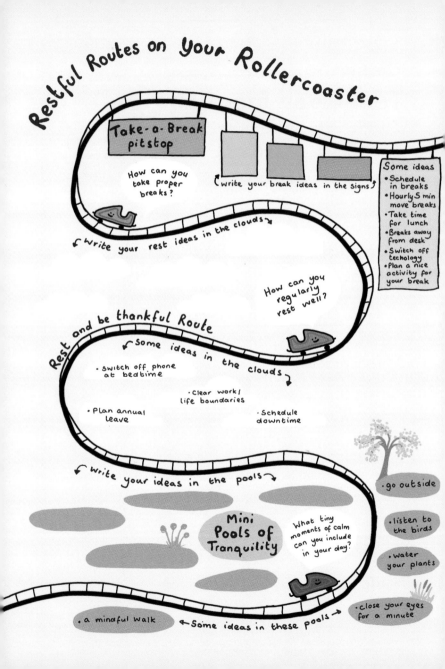

Soothing emotions

Let's focus on those sensations that sit at the bottom-right of the feelings compass and feel pleasant and soothing or de-energized. The labels we use to describe these states tend to be calm, peaceful, gentle and relaxed. The feelings you associate with these emotions might differ, but for many they will sit on the pleasant-sensation side of the compass. They are a key part of our emotional rollercoaster, looking after our mind and keeping our body budget in balance. However, life is busy, with endless demands. We rush, we plan, we tick off our to-do lists in our quest to get through the constant demands and tasks that life asks of us. This never-ending stream can result in an 'up-regulated' state of vigilance, as our brain tries to help us deal with these demands. Often, we stay in this up-regulated state for too long, chronically stressed. More pressure builds, as we forget to take breaks or do things that relax us.

Feeling calm and other soothing emotions are important pit stops to slow down your rollercoaster and help it function well. These emotions give your brain a break – helping you to relax, digest, heal and regulate stress, and contribute towards a healthy, happy body and mind. In short, they help you cope with the inevitable stressors that life throws at your rollercoaster.

Calm

It sounds simple doesn't it, to just relax, take it easy? If anybody has ever told you to 'just calm down' (especially when you're angry), you'll probably recognize how hard this is to do on demand. Getting your body to create those feelings of calm isn't always easy, and it can look different for each individual. In addition, there's all that debris that blocks the track to contend with as we direct our rollercoaster towards calmer stretches of track – digital distractions, brain distractions, societal expectations, and the belief that relaxation is indulgent or lazy. Yet, creating calm by taking relaxing breaks has been shown to reduce stress, increase energy and improve cognition, helping us manage our body budget effectively and positively impacting our bodies, mind and the resulting emotions we feel.

Connected

Feeling connected can be about linking to people who we feel understand, support and nurture us, or it might be connecting over common interests and values or towards a shared purpose. We can also feel connected to what's important to us on an individual level (our interests and ideals) through what we do and activities we take part in. Emotions can direct us to meaningful elements we want to connect more with in our lives. But how we feel can also be an important indicator that our values are being transgressed, or that we are not meeting our needs or values. Feeling connected in a meaningful way feels good because it produces positive affect, helps reduce stress, manages our body budget and is one of the strongest factors that improves health and wellbeing.

Contained

Feeling contained is feeling safe, heard and supported to express yourself and your emotions. On an individual level, the interconnectedness of our brains means the people we talk to and interact with strongly influence how we feel, because of how they regulate our nervous system and the affect this creates. People who make us feel contained are those who give us permission to feel. This validation is important for helping us process our emotions, and for regulating and channelling them so we can cope with difficult situations. It can untangle our difficult thoughts and help shift perspective. However, feeling contained doesn't always involve a deep dive into your emotions; it can just be about how people make you feel when you are with them.

Being the container can also be beneficial, as helping others makes us feel good. It's important to balance the amount you contain for others with how much you are contained yourself. We all need containers, but it may not be easy to trust someone, especially if you have had difficult past experiences. Sometimes, it's simply about finding the right people, and sometimes it's about learning to trust to be able to be contained, which is the basis of therapeutic relationships. It can be worth considering if this is a good place to start, if you find this emotion difficult.

Compassion

When we are compassionate and understanding of other people, it helps with their emotions and has a positive effect on how they feel. It also helps us, as it can reduce stress and create feel-good affect. Experiencing compassion towards yourself, either through other people (it's a part of being contained) or yourself is like wrapping your difficult emotions in a warm, cosy blanket and giving them a hot chocolate. It doesn't necessarily make them go away, but it soothes them and makes them feel less difficult to bear. Yet our natural response to ourselves is often the opposite of a warm blanket – we kick our emotions when they are down, setting our rollercoaster off on a downward trajectory, making our brain and body feel stressed and creating even more difficult emotions. We get stuck in difficult emotions rather than navigate through them. Compassion helps us navigate and understand *why* we are feeling bad, as well as accept those feelings. It also has a soothing effect on our physiology – compassion gives us a calming hug, which lowers the heart rate and dampens the body's stress response. We can nurture the power of compassion to create different feelings, leading to different emotions, helping us cope with life stressors and setbacks.

Restful routes on your rollercoaster

Think about the last time you felt calm. What was happening? Who was with you? Working out what makes you calm can help your rollercoaster run more smoothly. It can be about creating these feelings of calm in your body directly (through breathing, moving, etc.) or via your context and what you do (being in an environment that makes you feel safe). Including small pockets of calm, along with effective breaks and regular relaxation, will do wonders for you. Use the image on page 120 to think about how you can help your rollercoaster pass through the small pools of daily tranquility, meander regularly along the rest-and-be-thankful track or stop at the take-a-break pit stop.

When do you feel most connected?

Think about which people, values and activities make you feel connected, and note them below. Do you need more of these on your rollercoaster route?

People I feel
connected with

Activities I feel
connected with

Values I feel
connected with

Identify your containers

Having regular containment is important in both your professional and personal life. You can create this at work through peer support, mentoring, supervision or even just a lunch or coffee with your containers. In your personal life, you can spend time with those who contain you and reach out to them when you need support. Who are your containers? Who makes you feel secure and able to safely hold your emotions? Use the image below to think about your containers. Do you need to add anything to your rollercoaster route to ensure you feel contained more often?

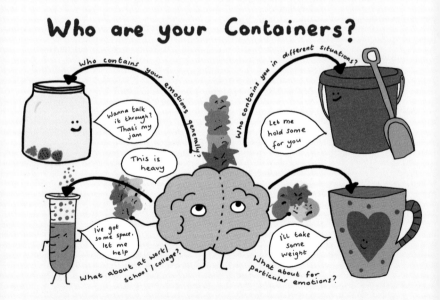

Give your heart a hug

Compassion is a win-win for your emotional rollercoaster, and you can be an active participant in creating this emotion. Don't be a heartbreaker, be a heart-hugger! Use the image below to recognize tendencies that break your heart, and remind yourself of ways to soothe your heart (and emotions) with the power of compassion.

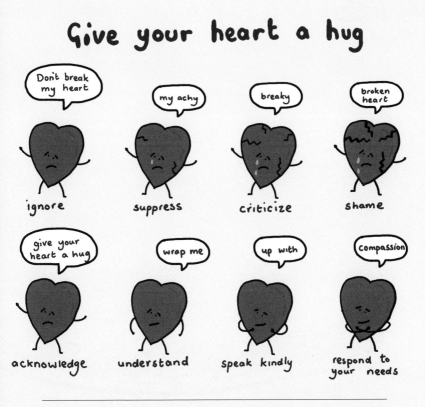

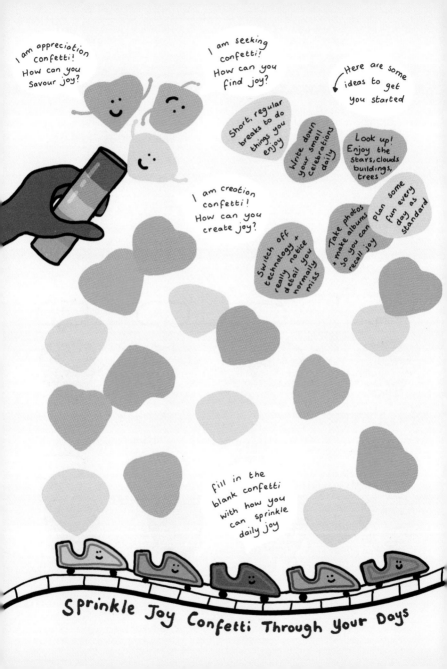

Upbeat emotions

We're now moving your rollercoaster to the top-right quadrant of the feelings compass to meet the emotions that we associate with feeling energized and upbeat. Remember, though: emotions are neither good nor bad; they all serve a purpose. Emotions are also unique, which means some I describe might feel different to you. They might even exist in a different place on your feelings compass. In addition, emotions often sit alongside one another. We don't experience them as a linear conveyor belt, one coming after the other; they come at us in pick-and-mix bags, often with contradictory emotions in the same bag. For example, love for your children can come with anxiety; excitement may come with fear; grief with relief; looking through old photos can be both wonderfully and sadly nostalgic.

While the emotions we discuss here are ones that we often hope to create on our rollercoaster route, in certain circumstances they may not be helpful. Let's take anticipation as an example. This is a result of our brain system getting ready for what it views as a reward, which floods our brain with dopamine, which makes us feel good, so that we work towards the end goal. Yet that very same system is the one that tech companies exploit so you anticipate the reward of likes, comments or new posts, and continue to scroll constantly through their TV channels, websites and social media, which can end up making you feel crappy. We can also use these feel-good hits to avoid difficult emotions, for example eating to mask emotions, or getting an exercise fix to avoid having to recognize sad feelings. The key is to understand how we can use these emotions along our rollercoaster ride to our benefit and create these emotions in a way that helps us feel good, without using them to negate or avoid the bad. Let's start by meeting joy.

Joy

An essential emotion on your rollercoaster ride, joy is about feeling pleasure or happiness. It makes you feel good, has a positive impact on health and wellbeing, and might even make you do good (research suggests you become more compassionate, open-minded and understanding when joyful). We can create joy, find it in what is already there or expand it by giving it some attention. Joy can be elusive – the brain can pass quickly over things that bring us joy, shifting to the next thing or becoming distracted by the negative. If we try too hard to seek it, making joy the end goal of whatever we do, it can dissipate. If we force ourselves to be joyful ('Hey, don't worry, be happy!'), it can evaporate under the pressure. If we use joy as a form of avoidance, ultimately it will be engulfed by other emotions as they pop back up. Joy would much rather you enjoy the ride while you're on it, rather than trying to reach a destination of joy at the end of the route. Joy can only ever pop up for short periods on the journey because all the other emotions need some space on the ride, too. Yet, joy doesn't like to be put on pause, nor does it believe you should wait for it; it thinks it should be an important and regular part of your journey. We tend to push joy away when times are hard, but it can be found lurking even at the darkest times, if you recognize it and let it in. Joy likes to be sprinkled through your day and along your journey like confetti, which you can create, find and appreciate.

Anticipation

We've already started to create anticipation with our joy confetti. Planning small pockets of joy in your day has a double whammy for how you feel – not only do you experience the (hopefully) positive affect, but you also have a build up to the event itself, which your brain anticipates, and which can impact on how you feel. Anticipation is a fundamental emotion of your predictive brain, and to get to know it better, you'll need to first meet your brain's reward system. This system is designed to help you survive, whether that be through finding food, a partner, sex, comfort or a nice cup of tea. To do this, it anticipates that these rewards will be good, activating a 'dopaminergic response', which drives your behaviour to seek the rewards and uses your memory to anticipate them in the future.

Yet, the anticipation of reward may turn out to be even more satisfying than the event itself, because your brain's reward system is activated even more when seeking and anticipating – compared to finding – the reward. This anticipation may drive your behaviour to seek a reward, even when it isn't good for you or is even unhelpful. I'm sure we can all think of a time when anticipation has gone wrong for us – chasing that elusive love interest when we know they would not be good for us, using social media to gain likes that don't actually make us feel good, or anticipating Friday-night drinks that actually wreck our weekend because of the inevitable hangover. The reward system has a hand in developing substance and behavioural addictions, as it creates that anticipatory craving that drives us to seek more of a substance or behaviour. While anticipation is a powerful and necessary feeling, its propensity to drive our behaviour in unhelpful directions stems from it feeling good. However, we can use this knowledge to create anticipation helpfully and navigate our rollercoaster ride.

Awe

Let's welcome awe to widen our perspectives, recognize the amazing world we live in and appreciate how small and interconnected we all are. Awe can mean the largeness of the universe or the smallness of an intricately shaped stone taking your breath away. Awe can take you outside of your mind and make you see things from a wider viewpoint. In doing so, awe also shrinks how big you feel: by shifting perspective outside your mind, you feel smaller in the world.

But this smallness is not about shrinking you as a person; it can make worries feel smaller, your everyday seem less troublesome, while also growing your worth and broadening your understanding and thinking. Awe has a hand in creating positive mood and reducing stress. We often use our eyes to experience the awe of landscapes, skyscapes and microcosms of the world, and there's fascinating research that indicates shifting our visual focus outwards into this panoramic mode reduces the physiological stress response. That's one good reason to put your phone down and shift your eyes from a narrow focus to the landscape next time you take a break.

Pride

Poor pride gets a bad press – as the saying (or myth) goes, 'pride comes before a fall'. Often, it's associated with having a big ego, arrogance or feeling superior to other people, which means our pride gets hidden as we mask our achievements and gloss over our successes. Ironically, we end up feeling ashamed of feeling proud. But, for me, pride is not about feeling that we are better than others, it's about recognizing our achievements: that we are just as good as others, that we all have daily struggles to overcome, that we are constantly riding the rollercoaster and navigating tough times and emotions. Pride means we can celebrate everyday success, not to the detriment of others but to the benefit of ourselves. Compassion may be the antidote to shame, but I see pride as the opposite of shame, if we use it to shift the situations that made us feel bad and see them through a new lens: 'I shouldn't be feeling this way' becomes 'I managed to get through the day despite feeling terrible'; 'I really mucked up in that presentation' becomes 'I managed to continue giving my talk even after I lost my place'. We need to feel pride not just for the good stuff, but also for overcoming challenges. Pride is not arrogance; it's giving yourself recognition for what you have managed, because life can be tough, and we should be proud of how we continue to travel along our rollercoaster route despite all the bumps, breaks and falling rocks. So, let's take pride out of the shadows and feel it in our achievements and challenges – and even take pride in feeling proud. In the words of Heather Small from M People, 'What have you done today to make you feel proud?'

Sprinkle joy confetti

What does joy mean to you? What brings you joy? Are there places you can create joy where you wouldn't naturally expect it (such as at work)? Can you allow yourself small pockets of joy when times are tough? Use the image on page 128 for ideas for sprinkling a handful of confetti during your rollercoaster ride. There are three types of joy confetti: creation, appreciation and seeking. Allowing time for each of these in regular, even tiny, moments in your day can impact positively on how you feel.

Creation confetti is about *planning* things you enjoy. A walk outside at lunchtime, a laugh with a friend, a tea break with colleagues. Whatever brings you joy, plan small pockets of it. Don't pressure yourself to feel joy (or else it might want to hide from you), just do the things you normally enjoy and see how they feel on any particular day, which may be different from another day.

Appreciation confetti is about taking time to *think* about the joy you've experienced. Our mind tends to pass over joy, so taking time to appreciate it can help extend and consolidate it in our memory. Consider what brought you joy today – what did you do well, what experiences lit you up? Look through your photos, write it down, tell someone about it, reminisce – all this expands joy.

Seeking confetti is about *noticing* what creates joy around you. What flowers are blooming on your walk? What funny antics are your pets up to today? What is changing in your children today? Notice this, take photos, cast it into memory – all this helps create further handfuls of joy confetti.

Anticipation creation

We all plan to some extent, but often it's the day-to-day chores we feel we must get done. Planning things to look forward to, in addition to the daily confetti, whether it be fun, relaxing or exciting activities, can help us create anticipation for positive events. This can increase the positive feeling of the event itself, through the double whammy of the anticipation as we think about the future event. In fact, get out your diary, look at tomorrow, next week, next month and see what positive events you have planned (if you're like me, you'll probably have multiple feel-good things planned for your kids but will have neglected your own calendar). Now, add some ideas – make time and space for creating feel-good emotions in the future as well as creating them in the present. Don't just plan what you *have* to do, plan what you want to do and enjoy. By doing this, you actively invite anticipation into your diary and allow it to impact positively on your rollercoaster.

Create awe

Use the prompts below to look at ways you can create awe in your daily life. You can also add awe to your exercises for anticipation-creation, joy-confetti or routes-to-relaxation in this chapter.

• What does awe feel like to you?

• What creates a sense of awe or wonder for you?

• How can you notice the things that make you feel this way (e.g. remove distractions, focus on the environment)?

• How can you incorporate awe into your days?

Put pride in its rightful place

Consider your beliefs about pride. You can use Exercise 1 on page 79, where we examined beliefs about emotions, to help with this. Do you feel you shouldn't be proud or that you should hide your achievements? How does this impact on your behaviour? Would you rather tell people all the things you've done wrong than what has gone well? Now, let's start to give pride the attention it deserves. It can be nice to do this exercise regularly, perhaps as part of the end-of-the-work-day routine. You may wish to do this with someone else, as it takes practice to let people know what you are proud of. Ask yourself these questions:

• What have I done today to make me feel proud?

• Have I faced any challenges today that I can be proud of? Has anything gone wrong today that I can be proud of my response to?

• Am I proud of how I responded to anyone else today?

• What can I do tomorrow that I will be proud of?

• When I look at where I was last year, what do I feel proud about?

• If I was looking at my situation from someone else's perspective, what would they tell me to be proud of?

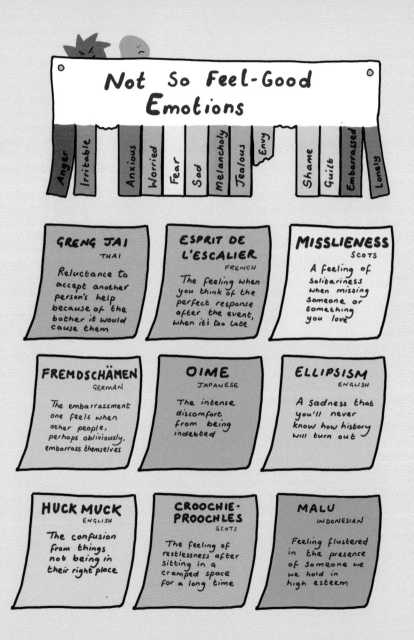

Chapter 5
Not So Feel-Good Emotions

Now we're moving along on our rollercoaster to those emotions that fall on the unpleasant side of the compass: the dips of sadness; the escalations of anxiety that can feel out of control; the overwhelm dead ends that we struggle to find a way out of; the troughs of guilt; the shame that seeps over the tracks; and the anger volcanoes that appear quickly, and sometimes out of nowhere. These bumps, troughs and escalations are an inevitable part of the rocky rollercoaster ride of life, and we need to understand and learn to ride through them. Depending on what we do, our responses to tough emotions can get us stuck in emotional ruts or help us navigate a way through them. You may think this chapter is going to take you into the chasm of doom, but actually, looking at these emotions and understanding our responses is a hopeful highway. By recognizing them as a normal part of life, we start to see them in a different light. Not the prophets of doom but indicators, prompts and signals that we can use to guide our behaviour and the future path of our rollercoaster in a beneficial direction. Of course, there are many more difficult emotions than those captured in this chapter, but many of the exercises used here and in Chapter 3 can be applied to help navigate them.

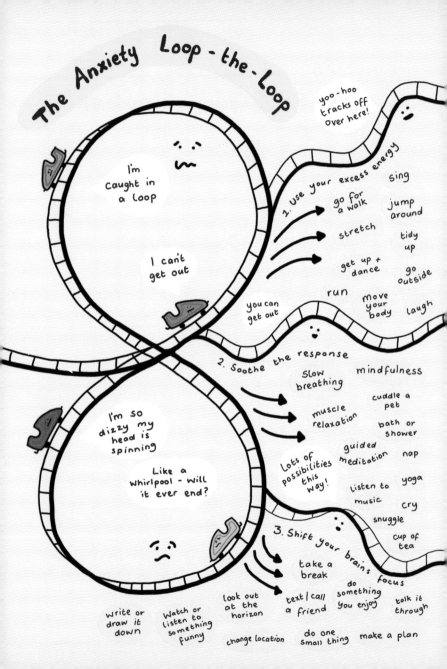

Anxiety and fear

Anxiety is a label we use to describe many body and mind responses, such as the content of our racing thoughts or our stomach churning away. How anxiety manifests in us, and therefore how we experience it, can vary widely – nerves, angst, worry, fretting, fear, panic. We might feel anxious in certain situations and label this as social anxiety. Or we might feel anxious in response to certain objects and label this as phobia. Anxiety is many different things to lots of different people, but many of us will understand or have experienced some version of it.

Nearly everyone will feel anxious when experiencing traumatic situations or major life stressors – it's to be expected. I'm sure every sports person will have experienced anxiety before an event. If you ask people about to take an exam, most will describe feeling anxious. If I was to host an imaginary anxiety party with Beyoncé, Michelle Obama, Tim Peake, David Attenborough and Bill Gates on the guest list (hey, aim high!), I'm pretty sure they could all describe a time when they'd felt anxious. Anxiety, and its conceptual friends worry and fear, are common emotions that vary in frequency, intensity and duration. We may think anxiety gets in the way of life, but it is designed to be helpful – to spot a threat and prepare you for action, to drive you towards or away from things that arise along your rollercoaster route. Anxiety can help you to spot when things are going wrong and flag when you have more stressors than capacity. However, the bodily response that is often at the root of the feelings we label as anxiety is also fundamental to our lives more generally.

Anxiety is associated with the flight-fight-freeze response: our body getting us ready for action based on our brain's predictions, so it can deliver the correct energy and bodily resources. At its root, this is about basic brain function, homeostasis, keeping your body in balance and using resources wisely. We know this is happening perpetually in our body as a required response for whatever we need to deal with, be that finding food, coping with a bully, being alert to meet a work deadline or even just getting up to face Monday morning. To do this, your brain triggers signals that release the hormones cortisol and adrenaline, engaging your sympathetic nervous system. This is the bodily response that can sometimes result in the feelings associated with anxiety: glucose is released into your blood stream and fat is broken down to give you energy; breathing increases to get more oxygen in your body; your heart beats faster to pump blood faster; your pupils dilate; your thinking becomes more focused; your senses sharpen; your muscles tense. All this gets your body ready to respond to whatever action is required, and your brain prioritizes its functions accordingly. This means it deprioritizes other more complex functions that might stop it achieving its goals: it inhibits digestion, more complex thinking and planning and saliva production (dry mouth, anyone?), and even narrows your visual field. While these types of body responses may result in a label of anxiety, they are not just about anxiety or fear, but are also about enabling you to live your day-to-day life effectively and use your energy to meet your needs. Engaging your sympathetic nervous system is a necessary part of staying heathy, safe and alive.

Sometimes, though, our predictions are out of kilter with our needs. The resulting revving up of our body systems can be detrimental to how we feel and our health longer term, as it throws our body out of balance. Our brain can over-predict threat for many reasons. We might be living through a stressful situation, so are already on high alert, with our brain primed for predicting threat. If we've experienced past trauma or stress related to a particular situation, our brain is likely to respond in a similar way when faced with a similar circumstance, and this might occur even when it spots similarities in seemingly insignificant data such as smells or noises. A history of high stress and trauma can also lead to developed brain pathways that are more likely to be vigilant to the possibility of threat. This is why even minor similarities in the incoming data can set off a huge bodily response. It might seem out of context, but your brain is telling you that based on past experience, you *need* to get ready for action.

When your brain predicts threat and gets your body revved up and your energy ready when you don't need it, that energy has nowhere to go and can stick around like an unwanted guest, creating the affect that we might label as 'anxiety'. This places huge demand on your body budget and can make you feel exhausted, tired, jaded and low, and can have implications for your health and wellbeing.

Our brains can also make sense of a physical sensation by labelling it anxiety, when there may be other reasons for what is going in. It's not unheard of for an underlying stomach or heart condition to be labelled as anxiety because the feelings they create are similar. If you are concerned that any anxiety symptoms may have an underlying cause, please get them checked by a medical professional.

Our response when anxiety strikes can either help us ride the anxiety wave or get us into a loop-the-loop that's difficult to exit. Anxiety doesn't feel nice, so it's natural to try to bury it, but avoidance means we don't deal with the problem. It also means we can never help our brains learn to make better predictions. For example, we may avoid social situations because we believe people won't like us. We can't disprove this theory if we never test the situation, so our beliefs stay the same. Some of our subtler actions are also a form of avoidance – the need for a drink to enable you to go out socially, seeking perpetual reassurance, or making extensive plans for how you will deal with the thing you're scared of. Although these actions may seem to reduce anxiety short term, long term they increase it. None of these things are inherently bad, but they can become unhelpful coping strategies if they are your go-to responses to anxiety.

When to label something as unhelpful avoidance is not always an easy decision to make. Is it helpfully reducing your mental load when required or is it unhelpful avoidance? While facing up to your fears to help your fears might sound ridiculous, it's backed up by sound scientific evidence. If you avoid something you are afraid of, your brain will continue to create feelings that you label as anxiety. However, if you gradually get used to something you are afraid of, your predictions will change and the resulting anxiety will gradually reduce. As a result, your brain will eventually realize it is making a prediction error and correct itself with new predictions.

Other things feed into the anxiety loop-the-loop, too. When our brain's predictions are out of kilter with our needs, the response created can keep us hooked in the emotion. Body reactions – our energy release, shallow breathing and racing heart – have nowhere to go, and are not used as our brain intended them to be, so we get stuck in them and they grow rather than reduce, making us more anxious. These exercises focus on finding ways to break the loop-the-loop of anxiety.

Routes through anxiety

Which routes can you use to get through anxiety and give your brain and body response somewhere helpful to go? Use the image on page 140 to help notice the signs you are stuck in a loop-the-loop, and think about which tracks could help you move through it. You can use more than one track.

Face your fears

Think about anything you are avoiding and use the image below to consider how you could gradually face this fear and help your brain to make better predictions.

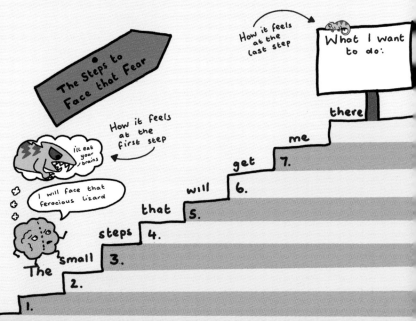

Get in your hot air balloon

The flight-and-fight response intentionally narrows your focus, both physically, through your eyes, and cognitively, through your brain processes and resulting thinking. This is helpful when needed but can become unhelpful when not. This exercise shows how you can widen your perspective, based on an analogy by Yale emotions researcher Marc Brackett featured on Dr Rangan Chatterjee's podcast.

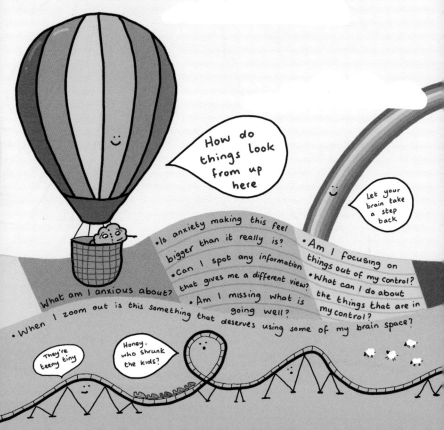

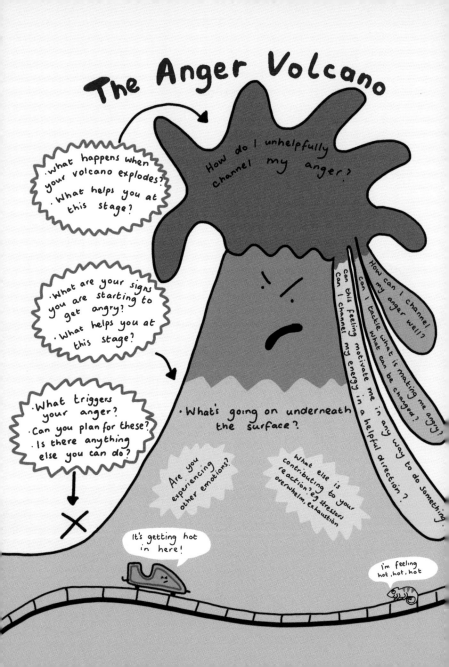

Anger

How does anger show up on your rollercoaster? Is it a giant volcano that emerges rapidly, wreaking destruction, derailing your cart or stopping you in your tracks? Is it a frustration that gets pushed down and bubbles under the surface until it bursts out, sometimes at random over something that wouldn't normally bother you? Does it arise in a wave of overwhelm in a work meeting? Is it the dominant way you express other emotions, such as disappointment, hurt and embarrassment? Does it come out only behind a screen, either in your car or when online? Maybe you've been told anger is something to be ashamed of so you've tucked it so far away you feel its distant echo at times but don't really know what you are feeling. The feeling might even be similar to other emotions, such as anxiety, as often similar physiological mechanisms underlie them, but we tend to label and understand anger differently. Of course, it could be all of these things, because anger is not a catch-all term; it includes multiple possible reactions and sensations with a variety of possible causes and consequences.

Now think about what causes anger. It can often arise as a response to unfairness – on your rollercoaster ride you feel you are being disrespected or undermined, and suddenly a sharp trajectory appears ahead and you accelerate up this unexpected anger rise at Lewis Hamilton pace. You might feel at risk, or that someone or something you care about is at risk and requires protection. Maybe it's caused by observing a strongly held value being transgressed. On my rollercoaster, one thing guaranteed to set off that volcano eruption is someone parking in a disabled spot unnecessarily. I feel it's extremely selfish and it pushes my anger button big time. Of course, the brain doesn't really have an anger button. It's creating these sensations through its predictions, and you create your emotions through your understanding of these feelings in the context you are in. In many instances of anger, your brain is predicting that you need energy to deal with whatever injustice, transgression or risk is coming your way.

Anger may also be the feeling and reaction that comes out when we are experiencing other emotions, particularly if we are trying to keep them contained or don't have ways to express them. It may be that hurt, disappointment, shame or embarrassment underlie your foaming reaction. Like the head of foam on top of a beer, this can overflow because there's too much going on underneath it that forces out the foam. If we are going through tough times, feeling other big emotions or experiencing too much pressure, our foam might erupt even at a tiny thing, which can seem strange if we don't understand what's going on underneath the foamy surface. We are also more likely to have outbursts of anger if we are already up-regulated: excited at a sports match, completed high-intensity workouts, under extreme pressure, or even very hot. It's well-documented that domestic violence incidents escalate during sports matches, which may be because people are already up-regulated with big feelings, making them more likely to respond with anger. Add alcohol, which reduces inhibition, and it can be a toxic mix. Inhibition can also be reduced by our context – being with a group of people acting the same, being behind the wheel of a car or being online all seem to reduce it. As a result, our brain seems to be more likely to issue predictions that result in feeling or expressing anger. How often do we see behaviour online that we would be far less likely to see in real life?

How we express, suppress or channel anger can become unhelpful. Our brain's predictions can be out of kilter with the context, based on past experience and what else is going on in our lives. Sometimes we get angry and we can't work out why. Sometimes our expectations are unrealistic (of both ourselves and other people) and we get angry when these standards are inevitably not met. Our beliefs about anger could lead us to suppress it if we view it as unacceptable, or, conversely, they might push us to express anger because we consider it a dominant and acceptable emotion (traditionally in men – research suggests that boys and girls are socialized to express their anger differently from a young age, with more overt expressions in boys). If we hold in what annoyed us during the day but then it comes out in excessive shouting and swearing when we get home, it can impact negatively on our relationships. If we're experiencing high stress or our defences are down, such as when sleep deprived, then we may become irritable and angry as a result. We are already up-regulated, and it doesn't take much to push that foam out of the glass, leading to behaviour that is out of character or of which we're not very proud.

Of course, anger isn't all bad. Many positive changes in the world have been driven by anger at injustice, discrimination and unfairness. Rosa Park's anger about racial discrimination led her to sit on that bus and not move. Greta Thunberg's anger at climate change drives her environmental campaigns, which impact positively on the world. Anger can give us the energy and momentum to ultimately improve the world that future generations of rollercoasters will ride through.

Anger often leads to secondary emotions. We might feel shame at experiencing anger, because of our beliefs about anger or embarrassment for how we've acted. We might feel regret for what we've said or done. This might lead us to mask anger in the future, which might work occasionally, but it's likely to slip out at some point when we have less cognitive resources to inhibit it. Ultimately, when you experience anger it's best to notice the factors underlying it, and find ways to understand and channel your anger well. In fact, getting to know your anger might just change your world, and the world as a whole, for the better.

What's fuelling your anger volcano?

Use the image on page 148 to help you think about what sets off your volcano eruption. Knowing what triggers your anger can help you to plan proactively for situations. Note down the signs that you are starting to get angry and think about strategies that might help. Use simple strategies when your volcano erupts, as your mind is overloaded so can't manage anything complex. Calm the physical response: breathe in slowly for three and out for four. Step out of the situation; use up your energy with quick bursts of physical activity – even shout and scream somewhere safe if it helps.

The lava at the top

Often, anger emerges when lots of other stuff is going on, or it can be an expression of other emotions. Digging down beneath the lava can help identify what needs to be tackled. Use the image on page 148 to think about what's happening under the surface.

The anger channel

You can't always stop anger arising, but you can think about how to channel it effectively. Use the questions in the image on page 148 to consider how you can move your anger to a helpful channel.

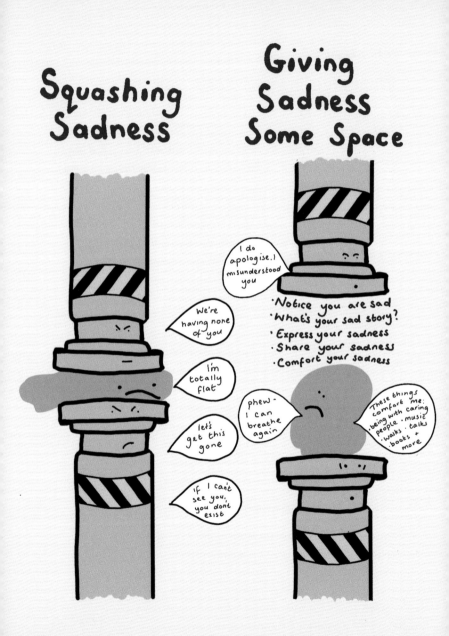

Sadness

Find me a person who has never felt sad and I will be hugely surprised. Sadness is such an integral part of the human experience that the nature of it (as helpful or a hindrance) has been debated throughout history. Feeling blue, despair, grief and many other labels have become the constructs of emotions used to describe the inevitable feelings we experience as a result of the various rocks hurled at our rollercoaster. You could even say that experiencing sadness is ubiquitous in some form or another.

Sadness crops up in all sorts of places, through the expected rollercoaster rocks of grief, loss, suffering, pain, illness, stress and overwhelm. Yet it also crops up at unexpected times, when we think we should be feeling positive: birthday celebrations that remind us of the time that has passed; longed-for babies whose happy arrival is mixed with sadness at the reality of newborn life; a long-awaited retirement where freedom beckoned but is tarnished by the lack of routine. Sadness is usually used to describe a temporary emotion, however it can become a longer part of our lives through depression (although this is not always about being sad – it can also be feeling empty, a lack of hope or positive emotions, or a lack of emotions altogether). Recent epidemiological research suggests that many of us will experience a prolonged period of low mood in our lifetime.

So sadness is part of life, as our emotional brains stumble through an unpredictable and difficult world. We need to learn to be sad; however, often we don't know how to, or won't allow ourselves to.

I suspect it would be easy to find me a person who has pretended not to be sad when they actually are. That's one of the ironies of this emotion – it's such a common part of life yet we often deny its very existence. Perhaps because it seems to sit in direct opposition to the emotion many of us pursue: happiness. However, in reality, sadness and happiness are more closely aligned than we might think, and one does not negate the other. We can experience sadness with things that make us happy, and we can experience happiness even in the darkest moments of our lives. Believing that sadness is something that points to some internal failure – a lack of ability to cope or to live life well – can result in an adversity to experiencing sadness. In our search for only positive vibes, our core coping strategy might be to push sadness aside with busyness, achievement, forced positivity and even substances. If this resonates with you, it might be helpful to use Exercise 1 on page 79 to look specifically at your beliefs about sadness and bust any myths that get in the way. Trying to kick sadness off the rollercoaster doesn't tend to work well for us: it's cognitively effortful, creates stress and doesn't allow us to process and understand our emotion, or tackle what it's trying to signal to us. It keeps on popping up and is likely to expand and stick around for longer in an attempt to get you to notice it.

Another irony of sadness is the perception of its futility. Cultural messages imply that happiness is your choice (which implies blame for the opposite), and this may have fed into your beliefs about sadness. Do you view feeling sad as wallowing? That crying is pitiful and you shouldn't show the world your sadness? It certainly influenced my beliefs and behaviour when I refused to cry at sad films as a teenager. Ironically, crying releases endorphins that help us feel better. It might have even made me a bit cooler (or at least have people feel positively towards me), as other people usually empathize with vulnerability. Research indicates that experiencing sadness might even be helpful to us. Sadness can highlight something is wrong: it indicates that we might need to do something to help us cope with what's going on in our life. It can also be an emotion of connection, helping us to form bonds. When we see sadness in others, it can be a sign to support them through difficult times.

Sadness may also enable us to experience happiness, as we can only appreciate feeling joy through comparison with difficult emotions. Many people I've worked with have come through difficult times and found they connect more to what's meaningful to them. So, sadness might help us slow down our rollercoaster, and analyse what's going wrong, which may help us move forward.

Like all emotions, sadness is linked closely to what's going on in the body. Interesting recent research has looked at how it is linked to the immune system. I feel inextricably sad when ill, and it seems this may be related to the immune response the body produces. When unwell, the body produces inflammation to heal wounds, or responds to threats to its survival such as bacteria and viruses. However, one of the effects of this may be to slow our brain and body, which produces feelings including tiredness and wanting to withdraw, which we conceptualize as sadness. In evolutionary thinking, withdrawal not only lets you rest and recuperate, it may also be helpful to those around you by signalling that you need support, or by separating you from the tribe, thereby reducing the spread of infection. Chronic stress produces a similar immune response, which may be why we respond with burnout, exhaustion or low mood in these instances.

So, sadness may have a beneficial role, and believing this may help us to allow it into our lives, to give it space instead of pushing it away. How we respond to sadness, often driven by our beliefs about it, might help or make it more difficult for us. Masking our sadness means people don't know we need support. They can't help fix our rollercoaster's wheels if we are pretending they are still working. Often our response to sadness is driven by the impact of sadness itself. It provokes ruminative and negative thoughts designed to direct your attention to and solve the problem, but which hook us in and are difficult to move on from. Although these thoughts are a product of our mood, we blame ourselves for feeling the way we do, which only pushes us further into the sadness. Our brain becomes fixated on problems, and because flexibility and new learning is reduced, we can't see ways out of the sadness tunnel. Our future predictions are influenced by our mood, and we predict we will not enjoy things, so don't do them, which impacts our mood further. The very processes that sadness creates can push us further into the sad tunnel, sometimes even directing us into a black hole, where hope feels lost and we can't see any way to climb out. If you find yourself in that black hole, then professional help may be required. If you are worried about depression, please talk to a health professional about possible support and/or treatment.

These exercises are designed to help you navigate sadness on your rollercoaster ride. You'll notice that they are not trying to fix sadness, rather to enable it and consider how best to respond. We can't shut our eyes as we pass through melancholy meadows, under sombre skies or across despondent deserts and pretend it's not happening, because this makes the carriages more likely to get stuck. If we give this emotion the space it deserves, we are less likely to get hooked in its ways and more likely to find our way through.

Give sadness some space

Are there ways you try to crush your sadness? How can you give your sadness some space to breathe, and enable yourself to recognize, see and understand it? Use the image on page 154 to think about how you might do this.

Find points of light

Emotions are transient by their very nature. We can feel rubbish and still get joy from some pretty flowers or a funny joke. These are not incongruous, it's the nature of our constantly changing and mixed emotions. Difficult emotions can sit alongside positive emotions. However, when we feel bad, we sometimes need to give ourselves permission to spot and feel the good in the midst of how we are feeling. These points of joy, relaxation or laughter are important to help you get through tough times: they are little lights that can guide you through the sadness tunnel. When you are suffering, you may need to encourage your attention to find the good; things you can take pleasure in, even for short times. Spot the flowers blooming in your garden, hear your children laughing, enjoy a decent coffee in the sunshine, have a brief walk around the garden. Allow yourself to tune in to whatever makes you feel good, even just for a few short minutes. Your brain might be telling you not to, but you could find a tiny bit of meaning, pleasure or relaxation that provides a light to guide you through.

Tune in to tune out

When you feel sad, you are more likely to be self-critical, find fault or see the worst-case scenario. In her book *How to be Sad*, Helen Russell calls this her 'Shit FM'. We all have a Shit FM that our radio tunes in to when we're feeling sad – each will play slightly different music. Being aware of when your radio has tuned in to Shit FM can help you find ways to respond helpfully rather than believing what it says to you and letting it push you further into the sadness tunnel.

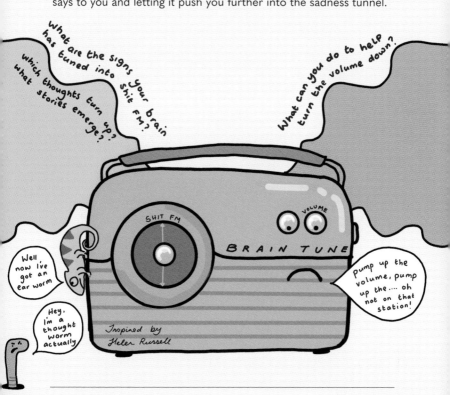

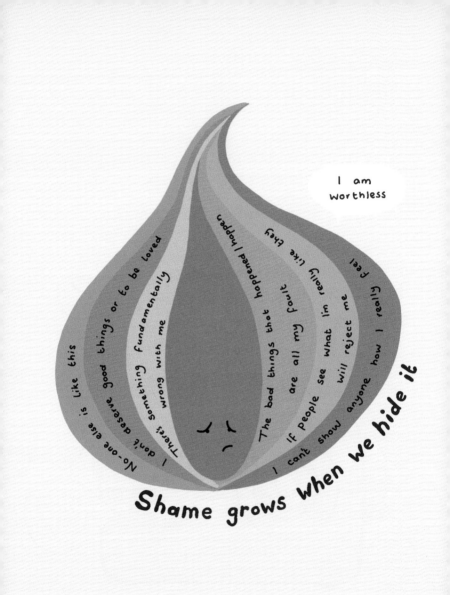

Guilt and shame

Guilt and shame can be thought of as pointers to tell us we have done something wrong that needs amending, that we have not done what we should have, or that we have not met either our own or others' standards or expectations. These emotions can help us to live within our values, and in a wider context create communities that function well. They can help us put our rollercoaster back on track when it's straying off course.

Sometimes these pointers go astray. Like a broken compass, they point to things we feel shame or guilt about when there's no reason to feel that way at all. We blame ourselves for things that we are not responsible for. We feel guilt when we fall short of the standards set by society, when really they are just not a good fit for us. Or we feel guilty when we try to live by an unrealistic set of 'shoulds' that no one could meet. Indeed, you may have been shamed by someone else about something, so you believe you are at fault or that you *are* the fault, leading to difficult emotions that grow beneath the surface where they can never be disproved. People can make us feel guilty about not meeting *their* unrealistic standards, and we work harder to try to meet them, to our detriment. You may have been ridiculed or bullied at school about a particular trait, which leads to a feeling of shame even though there's nothing inherently wrong with that trait.

As children, we are particularly vulnerable to internalizing and blaming ourselves for events when they are not our fault, and we can feel guilt or shame about this years later. They could be awful experiences such as abuse, or other difficult life events such as a parental divorce, where we were not responsible in the slightest but felt we were, and that feeling pervades into adulthood, especially when kept under wraps, where it thrives and grows.

Shame and guilt are often used interchangeably, along with words such as embarrassment and humiliation. How you conceptualize these might differ from other people, and there's a variety of different ideas of what these mean. I find Brené Brown's conceptualization helpful, which differentiates guilt and shame in the following way: guilt is about doing something wrong, 'I have made a mistake or done something bad'; shame is about you being wrong, 'I am a mistake or I am bad'. This is the conceptualization I am going to use when I speak about guilt and shame here.

Sometimes it can be helpful to have a guilty conscience, as it directs us to recognize when we are not meeting our values, hurting other people or doing something that we want to change. Feeling guilt can flag that we have broken our own, usually unwritten, code of conduct of who we want to be and how we want to act. However, sometimes we need to question the level of expectation we are setting, which can result in us feeling guilt not because we have got it wrong but because we *feel* we have got it wrong. If we set unrealistic expectations, feelings of guilt can become too frequent and unhelpful. They can also get in the way of us doing what is beneficial. The vague expectation that we should be doing more (which may have been set by a culture of productivity in this context), for example, means we can feel guilty when we take much-needed downtime or we end up saying sorry all the time, sometimes just for existing. The expectation we should do things perfectly is hugely unrealistic and will result in inevitable guilt, because we all make mistakes.

We also need to think about whose expectations we are striving to fulfil. Parenting is a good example. When we become parents, it sometimes feels as if we have a Guilt Fairy constantly telling us what we are doing wrong. This is partly helpful, because parenting is an important job after all and we want to try and get it right. But our Guilt Fairy can get out of hand quickly, criticizing us for nearly everything we do, when actually we are doing just fine, sometimes getting it wrong but learning, like every parent does. Our high expectations might be set by society, which says parents should be fully available, relaxed, calm and never shout, with children who behave at all times. We need to spot when our expectations have been set for us and decide whether we agree with these rules, or if they simply create false guilt.

Shame can be an insidious emotion that wreaks havoc when kept under cover. It grows when we hide the vulnerabilities we are ashamed of because we think sharing them may confirm what we believe: that we are fundamentally flawed and somehow different to other people. We may feel we are not worthy of love, undeserving of success, or not good enough to be in the job we're in.

While shame isn't inherently bad, we need to recognize what we are right to be ashamed of and seek to change our behaviour. In this way, shame has the ability to improve our lives and the lives of those who cross our path. However, facing up to justified shame is extremely difficult, even when it's directing us helpfully to take responsibility for our behaviour and actions. When we look inside ourselves and see things we don't like, we naturally want to avoid it and bottle it up; and that's why it can result in aggression, blaming others, addiction or mental health difficulties.

Often, though, shame points to things that are not our responsibility but that we think are, due to our experiences or what we've been told. This is often the case with abuse or bullying – we internalize it, making it something fundamentally about us as a person, leading to shame that we tuck away. Therapy is often required to uncover that shame and look at where the blame lies. Shame can also be driven by those same societal expectations that drive guilt: being the best mother, father, employee, wife; having the ideal house. Ultimately, shame is usually tied to our self-worth. We think we should behave a certain way, and when we don't we tell ourselves that something is wrong with us: we hide our vulnerabilities so we don't show the world our flaws. We may seek worth in things that are fragile, such as perfect homes or relationships and constant achievement. Yet these things are often unobtainable, and at the very least highly changeable, so we are likely to feel worse when they don't happen.

Shame is intrinsically linked to mental health. We feel ashamed for feeling bad, sad or worried, and this shame creates further difficult emotions and fuels poor mental health. This ties into the myths about emotions we talked about in Chapter 1: that we should be feeling fine all the time. This is not the case, as we *all* experience difficult emotions, and many of us will experience poor mental health at some point. An important part of improving mental health is reducing the shame people feel by exposing it, sharing it and letting others empathize.

Pulling shame out of the darkness and into the light shrinks it; you recognize you are not at fault, realize you are not different and discover collective experiences that validate your own. This can be scary, and it is a brave step that may need to be taken in a safe, clinical space in the first instance, if shame is strong or you have had very difficult experiences.

Peel back the layers of shame

This exercise looks at what expectations you are setting yourself and where you are placing responsibility, to think about how you could safely peel back the layers and get to the heart of shame. Compare the image on page 162 with the one below to help you consider this in more detail.

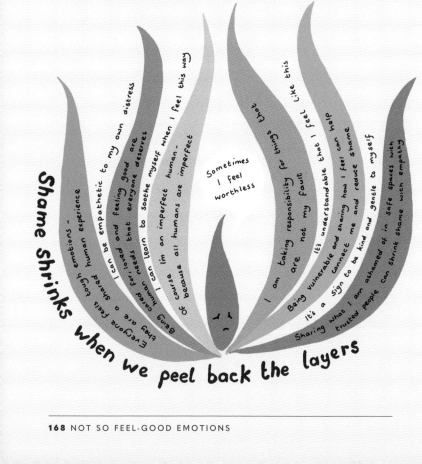

Shame shrinks when we peel back the layers

Everyone feels tough human emotions – they are a shared human experience

Being cared for and feeling good are human needs that everyone deserves

I can be empathetic to my own distress

I can learn to soothe myself when I feel this way

Of course I'm an imperfect human – because all humans are imperfect

Sometimes I feel worthless

I am taking responsibility for things that are not my fault

It's understandable that I feel like this

Being vulnerable and sharing how I feel can help connect me and reduce shame

It's a sign to be kind and gentle to myself

Sharing what I am ashamed of in safe spaces with trusted people can shrink shame with empathy

Fragile and stable self-worth

Shame is intrinsically linked to how we view ourselves and our self-worth. Self-worth is understanding that you have intrinsic worth and living in line with your own values rather than external expectations. Use the image to think about where you gain your self-worth from, and if there are ways to create greater self-worth by linking it to the more stable measures in the rocks instead.

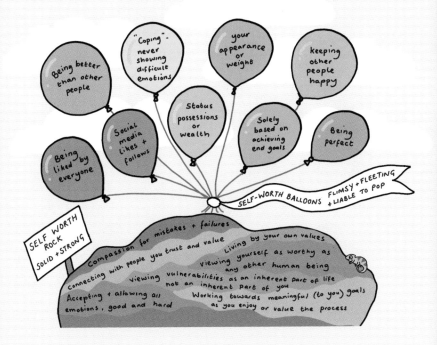

Being better than other people

"Coping" - never showing difficult emotions

your appearance or weight

keeping other people happy

Status possessions or wealth

Solely based on achieving end goals

Being perfect

Social media likes + follows

Being liked by everyone

SELF-WORTH BALLOONS FLIMSY + FLEETING + LIABLE TO POP

SELF WORTH ROCK SOLID + STRONG

Compassion for mistakes + failures

Living by your own values

connecting with people you trust and value

Viewing yourself as worthy as any other human being

Viewing vulnerabilities as an inherent part of life not an inherent part of you

Accepting + allowing all emotions, good and hard

Working towards meaningful (to you) goals as you enjoy or value the process

To guilt or not to guilt

Use this flowchart when you notice you are feeling guilty, to consider whether it's justified or if it's a false sense of guilt, and what they can do to help in these situations.

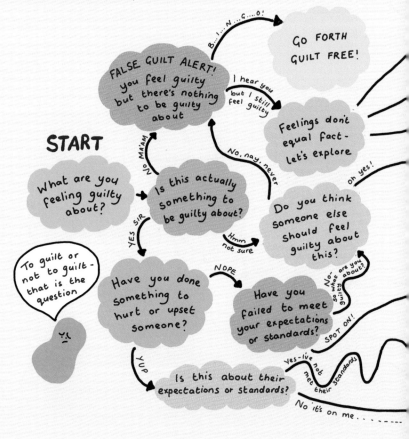

START

What are you feeling guilty about?

To guilt or not to guilt - that is the question

YES SIR

Is this actually something to be guilty about?

No MA'AM

FALSE GUILT ALERT! You feel guilty but there's nothing to be guilty about

B...I...N...G...O!

GO FORTH GUILT FREE!

I hear you but I still feel guilty

No, nay, never

Feelings don't equal fact - let's explore

oh yes!

Hmm... not sure

Do you think someone else should feel guilty about this?

No, so what are you guilty about?

Have you done something to hurt or upset someone?

NOPE

Have you failed to meet your expectations or standards?

SPOT ON!

YUP

Is this about their expectations or standards?

Yes - I've not met their standards

No it's on me...

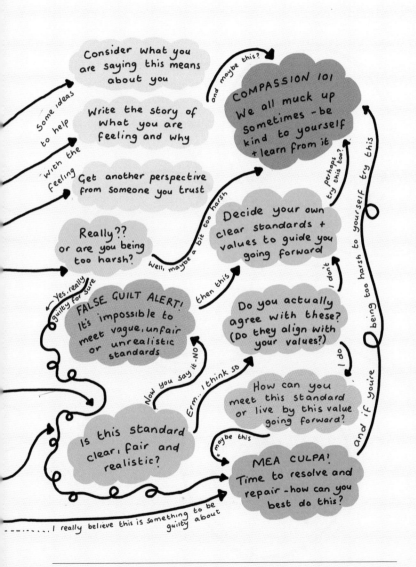

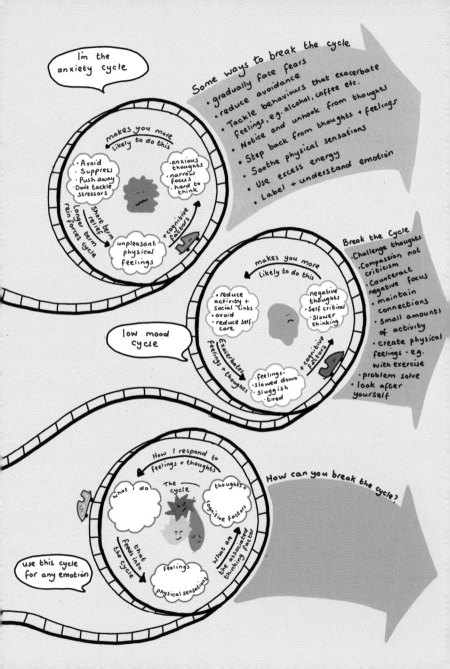

Chapter 6
Patterns in Emotions and Behaviours

What a rollercoaster we've been on so far, travelling through just some of the many emotions you might experience during your life and getting to know them better. Don't relax yet, though, because it's time for the final push to the end. This last bit of the track consists of some discombobulating loop-the-loops and stop/start gates as we look at how we can break patterns that don't serve us in our responses to emotions. We're also going to stop off at some junction points to see how we might take a slightly different trajectory, creating more of the emotions we want on our future rollercoaster. Plus, we'll be finding ways out of the tangled loop-the-loops we sometimes get stuck in. It's all about making and breaking emotional patterns, and we can't pretend this part of the journey is a breeze. It involves learning new skills and responses to soothe, navigate and create emotions. We're building new tracks for our rollercoaster to travel on and that takes time, energy and perseverance. But as we build these tracks, we'll find that our emotions start to become the helpful travel companions that they've always meant to be.

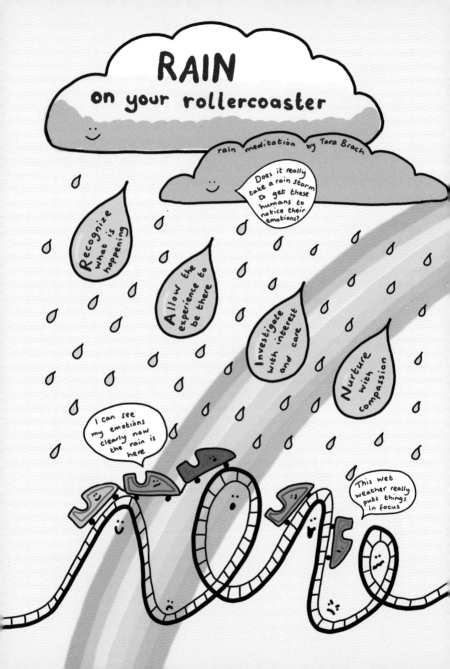

Making and breaking patterns

Roll up, roll up! Ready for some novelty? We're preparing to ride new routes on our emotional rollercoaster, going along lesser-travelled tracks, taking diversions and even building brand new tracks to travel along in the future. Building new routes and taking diversions asks more of the brain, as it needs to exert more effort to move off the well-travelled path and make new predictions. This is effortful at first, but gradually becomes easier and, eventually becomes a reflex. Making and breaking emotional patterns demands more of our body budget too, because it means moving away from our habitual track that's easy and smooth to ride along. We are going to focus on creating patterns of emotions (by building feel-good emotions into our day) and breaking patterns (by looking at patterns that get us stuck in unhelpful loop-the-loops).

Emotions are central to the task of taking new routes on our rollercoaster. If we beat ourselves up when we go astray or don't manage to do what we intended, this makes us feel bad and our brain associates this feeling with what we are doing, which makes it feel too difficult. We are more likely to give up or go back to our normal route, which, ironically, leads to feeling bad when we were trying to feel good. All of our rollercoasters inevitably deviate from our intended course, because that's just life, and we all need support to get back on the track we want to follow. Think of it like the effect of an onlooking crowd – if they berate and boo you when you don't manage, are you going to keep on trying? (We sometimes think negative self-talk or pressure pushes us on, but the evidence suggests that having this booing crowd just makes us feel rubbish and unmotivated longer term.)

Creating and breaking patterns needs to be supported by a crowd of cheerleaders, whether this be your own internal voice or the people in your life (or preferably both). These cheerleaders don't need to pretend that you are always fantastic, but they understand that you, like everyone else, won't always get it right. You are also likely to return to a well-worn but unhelpful track when your body budget is low, your brain is overloaded, or you are tired, stressed, overwhelmed or feeling bad. Instead of focusing on what went wrong, your cheerleaders need to understand why it's happening (if possible), that this is normal, and see if there's anything you can learn from it. It's also important that rather than shaming you and internalizing when it doesn't go right (it's all your fault, it'll never go right), they instead approach it with compassion, by speaking kindly to you while also calling out the story that some of the less supportive crowd (that negative self-talk) may be telling you. You need your cheerleaders to shout louder.

So, before we start making any changes, let's think about which supportive voices you want to cheer you on your way. Think of this in terms of what you tell yourself, but also think about who in your life forms the supportive crowd that will help you through any new routes you plan to take. Things seem more possible and manageable with support.

Creating patterns

We often want to help our emotions by doing something new, to create emotions that have a positive impact on how we feel. We may think this requires an overhaul, a huge U-turn or an entirely new path, but often it's the tiny tweaks of the steering wheel that set our rollercoaster off on a slightly different direction, which seem insignificant at first but longer term can lead to an entirely different path altogether. Small daily things – a short break, a mini walk, a healthy breakfast, an extra glass of water, a dose of joy, time to relax, a moment of awe – help manage your body budget and make you feel good; they're the ingredients for feel-good emotions. These daily tweaks may seem ridiculously easy, but they are often more likely to lead to long-term change than grandiose gestures. Why? It all comes back to emotions. The tweaks feel achievable, so we are more likely to start them, and starting is much of the battle; once we've begun something that feels good, we are much more likely to keep on going. This sense of achievement is intrinsically rewarding, and we want to do more. We just need to believe in the power of tiny tweaks to our trajectory, to create long-term impact on how we feel and our emotions.

Research also provides lots of evidence about how we can use our emotions to ensure we are more likely to keep going with any of our tiny trajectory shifts. Instead of berating ourselves for veering off track (it's inevitable, because our rollercoaster rarely travels in straight lines), we can create positive emotions by giving ourselves credit for what we *have* achieved. We can focus on the feel-good parts of the journey, rather than looking off into the distance towards an end goal. Enjoy the ride rather than focusing on the destination. Recording your progress in a positive manner and celebrating even tiny achievements will bring your attention to what you have done. And doing activities or recording progress with other people can give you even more of a positive boost. Combine things that you enjoy – a double feel-good whammy – meet a friend while walking, listen to music while exercising, for example.

Positive prompts can also build habits that are good for your emotions. This might be drinking water whenever you end a meeting, or prompting yourself to stop and take a rest at lunchtime by meeting a friend. Planning can also be a powerful tool: plan downtime and feel-good activities. If it's written down in black and white and you have already allocated time for it, you are much more likely to do it.

Changing the trajectory with tiny tweaks

Think about tiny tweaks you can use to build feel-good emotions into your day. A slight shift may seem insignificant, but over time it may take you on a totally different trajectory. What tiny tweaks can you add into your rollercoaster to change trajectory?

Your cheerleading crowd

Use the image below to consider what you want your crowd to tell you, to help you create positive change and also be compassionate when you veer off your intended course. Remind yourself of this when your critical crowd-voice grows louder.

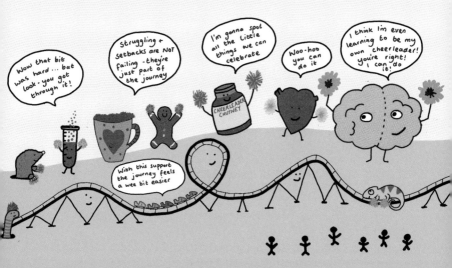

Breaking patterns

Building new pathways is part of looking after our emotions, but breaking old pathways and patterns we are stuck in is another. The tracks of our emotions can become habitual: our brain automatically predicts what will happen next and we follow suit, led into the same automatic responses that get us stuck in those tangled loop-the-loops that are difficult to navigate. Often these are age-old patterns that possibly developed at a time when they were helpful or served a function. As a child, you may have learned to avoid conflict within the family in order to keep yourself safe or not get into trouble, which has led to avoidance of anger or conflict as an adult. This means you get stuck, and never tackle or move on from these feelings. You may have learned to deal with anxiety by doing everything perfectly, being the good child who never did anything wrong, which worked until maintaining this perfect persona resulted in more anxiety than it solved, creating stress and demand on your body budget. We all have patterns, and it can be difficult to shift away from them, as they are automatic and habitual. Our brain's predictions mean we travel along these sections of track before we are even aware we are doing so.

You may also get caught in the loop-the-loop that certain emotions create by their very nature. You may have learned to manage your anxiety by avoiding what makes you feel bad, and this provides short-term relief but long-term discomfort.

Low mood makes you withdraw to keep you safe, but this ultimately makes you feel worse. All of us are prone to patterns that seem to keep us safe, but which, in some circumstances, have the opposite effect and make us feel worse.

The time when we most need to do something different is often when our emotions are difficult and our body budget most depleted, which means it can be even harder for the brain to break an old pattern or create a new one. So we need to use our best emotional tricks of the trade to help us, but be compassionate when we continue riding along the same rails.

It may seem like you're travelling with unstoppable momentum down a one-way track. However, the more you stop and change your response to your emotions then the more you build different tracks, ones that give you different options when the emotions occur and that mean you can step off onto another track. It may be overgrown and difficult to ride at first, but the more you use it, the more likely your brain is to predict that this track is the correct route, meaning the more likely you are to take it, and the smoother and easier the track will become for you to take in the future.

The first action in changing tracks is being aware that emotions are arising. Awareness acts as a slow-down sign on the track, indicating that we can stop and think, have agency about how we respond and decide to step off the habitual track onto a more helpful response route.

The following exercises will help you to slow down and create space between your emotions and the response, as well as identifying your own patterns, and small but effective changes to break them and forge new tracks.

RAIN on your rollercoaster

This exercise is based on Tara Brach's RAIN meditation and aims to increase awareness and allow you to step back from emotions so you can shift onto the tracks of your choice. Recognize, Allow, Investigate, Nurture: a nice acronym to use as a prompt to be aware of what's going on and think about where you want to go next on your track. Use the image on page 174 to consider the signs that you need to slow down and create RAIN on your rollercoaster, and think actively about where you would want to go next with this emotion, rather than being driven by your habitual emotion responses.

Breaking out of the loop-the-loops

What emotional pattern of response loop-the-loops do you get stuck in? The image on page 172 has specific loop-the-loops that are based on models of anxiety and low mood. However, you can use the ideas for any emotions with which you have difficulty. List some of the patterns you get stuck in and what could be the small intervention that could create different routes next time you experience those emotions. It is easier to spot loop-the-loops and plan new routes when you are feeling okay. Once you become aware you are feeling the emotion again, you can prompt your brain to take the new route instead of getting stuck.

Emotions:
The Ride Continues

The chequered flag is in sight and we've come to end of the track – and what an emotional journey it's been. We've baked some cookies, meandered to islands where negative emotions don't exist, been on dozens of loop-the-loops, predicted the future, time-travelled through history, dispelled lizards from our brains and perhaps even jettisoned some past beliefs from our rollercoasters. Our emotions have been constant companions on the ride, never left behind or rejected for being negative, but noticed, validated, understood, sieved, given space, labelled, soothed and used to help us navigate the ride.

It may be the end of our journey together through this book, but it's just the first step for your own journey. How will you move forward with your emotions as a central and inevitable part of your life? Perhaps you'll view them differently, as meaningful data rather than unwanted intrusions to your day. Perhaps when emotions show up, you'll start to notice them more, as they rise your shoulders with tension, make your head dizzy with anticipation or soothe you into calmness. Perhaps you'll accept them as travel companions, so they sit alongside you on your journey. You might even join my club and build your own collection of emotions, and in doing so expand your concepts and fine-tune your brain's predictions and understanding of what the heck is happening when those feelings arise. Whatever you do, in growing your emotional expertise you'll be putting emotions in their rightful place at the heart of your future rollercoaster, to help you navigate and build your track. Remember, though, that your brain will inevitably take you back on habitual routes, so keep referring back to your rollercoaster of relevant thoughts and ideas (see page 14) to remind you what you can do when emotions arise, to help understand, respond to and navigate them.

We also create emotions in others through our words and actions, as well as construct other peoples' emotions by trying to anticipate and understand how they feel. Our rollercoaster supports people we are connected to and holds them up when they are down, or contains or calms them when they are up. Our words hold power to inflict emotional damage or heal emotional pain. Our actions create and break emotions in others. Our emotional rides intersect, getting caught up with one another in tangled patterns that can be difficult to unwind. This interaction of emotions between brains also places responsibility on all of us for how we impact on others.

Whether by enabling discussions of how we feel at work or just in our day-to-day lives with family or friends, putting our emotions at the heart of what we do and how we interact instead of stifling or ignoring them has benefits for all of us. If we allow an understanding of emotions, even in environments where they aren't traditionally acknowledged (such as workplaces, schools, universities and civic spaces), it helps us tackle tricky situations, create better cultures, understand and identify issues and find solutions. The evidence shows us that giving emotions space and time helps us work better, learn better, connect better, innovate better, respond better, live better and, of course, feel better, in whatever situation we are in.

Our knowledge of emotions also brings responsibility for future generations. There have been generational shifts in how children are taught and speak about emotions, and that's a hugely positive thing. Enabling children to articulate how they feel, without punishment or minimizing feedback, helps children understand themselves and their needs as they ride through life. Creating an emotional vocabulary supports that understanding, and helps their brains guide them with more finely tuned and accurate predictions. Allowing space for their emotions gives children the confidence of knowing that they can feel bad yet get through it and learn what to do when they feel that way in the future. All this will help them make sense of the inevitable loop-the-loops they will have to navigate with their emotions by their side. I've included a number of resources in the Further Reading section (see page 188) if you want to look into this further.

I've experienced a lot of emotions as I wrote this book, and I'm sure you have experienced a lot of emotions while reading it. For me, some of them were about the book, but many were about everything else going on during my rollercoaster ride. I've come a long way since my teenage years, but I'm not always a model example for how I apply the theory and respond to my own emotions – we can all get overwhelmed with life before we notice it. We are all just emotional brains riding through life, trying to navigate the ups and downs, not always getting it right but doing our best. There's no doubt that emotions can be frustrating, overwhelming and downright annoying, but they are necessary and inevitable. So, let's give emotions the standing they deserve, because they are not add-ons, irrational guests, the soft and fluffy stuff or evolutionarily redundant. They are at the heart of what it means to be human.

Further Reading

You can find out more about some of the topics discussed in this book with these resources.

Some of my emotions collection came from: Koenig, John, *The Dictionary of Obscure Sorrows*, Simon & Schuster, 2022 www.dictionaryofobscuresorrows.com

Chapter 1: **Getting to Know Emotions**
Damasio, Antonio, *The Feeling Of What Happens: Body and Emotion in the Making of Consciousness*, Mariner Books, 2000

Cesario, J., Johnson, D.J., & Eisthen, H.L., 'Your brain is not an onion with a tiny reptile inside', *Current Directions in Psychological Science*, 29(3), 255–260, 2020

Mlodinow, Leonard, *Emotional: The New Thinking About Feelings*, Penguin, 2022

Beck, Julie, 'Hard Feelings: Science's Struggle to Define Emotions', The Atlantic, 24 February 2015

Kleinginna, P.R. & Kleinginna, A.M., 'A categorized list of emotion definitions, with suggestions for a consensual definition', *Motivation and Emotions*, 5(4), 345–379, 1981

Dixon, T., '"Emotion": The history of a keyword in crisis', *Emotion Review*, 4(4), 338–344, 2012

Darwin, Charles, *The Expression of the Emotions in Man and Animals*, John Murray, 1872

Sagan, C., *The Dragons of Eden: Speculations on the Evolution of Human Intelligence*, Random House, 1977

Ekman, P., 'An argument for basic emotions', Cognition and Emotion, 6(3–4), 169–200, 1992

Lisa Feldman Barrett's page and research: https://lisafeldmanbarrett.com

Barrett, L.F., 'The theory of constructed emotion: an active inference account of interoception and categorization', *Social Cognitive and Affective Neuroscience*, 12(1), 1–23, 2017

Barrett, Lisa Feldman, *How Emotions Are Made: The Secret Life of the Brain*, Pan Books, 2018

Barrett, Lisa Feldman, *Seven and a Half Lessons About the Brain*, Picador, 2021

Chapter 2: **Why We All React Differently**
Therapy for Real Life podcast, 'Understanding the Body Budget with Lisa Feldman Barrett' https://anchor.fm/therapy-for-real-life/episodes/Understanding-The-Body-Budget-with-Lisa-Feldman-Barrett--PhD-eljs7a

Chao, R.C-L., 'Managing stress and maintaining well-being: Social support, problem-focused coping, and avoidant coping', *Journal of Counseling & Development*, 89(3), 338–348, 2011

Elliott, R., Rubinsztein, J., Sahakian, B., & Dolan, R., 'The neural basis of mood-congruent processing biases in depression', *Archives of General Psychiatry*, 59(7), 597–604, 2002

For acceptance and commitment exercises on unhooking from thoughts, see Dr. Russ Harris' website, https://thehappinesstrap.com

Tseng, J. & Poppenk, J., 'Brain meta-state transitions demarcate thoughts across task contexts exposing the mental noise of trait neuroticism', *Nature Communications*, 11, 3480, 2020

Chapter 3: **Responding to Our Emotions**
David, Susan, *Emotional Agility: Get Unstuck, Embrace Change and Thrive in Work and Life*, Avery Publishing Group, 2016

Cameron, L.D. & Overall, N.C., 'Suppression and expression as distinct emotion-regulation processes in daily interactions: Longitudinal and meta-analyses', *Emotion*, 18(4), 465–480, 2018

Posner J., Russell J.A., & Peterson B.S., 'The circumplex model of affect: an integrative approach to affective neuroscience, cognitive development, and psychopathology', *Development and Psychopathology*, 17(3), 715–34, 2005

Dr. Laurie Santos' podcast, The Happiness Lab, with Brené Brown's quote: www.pushkin.fm/podcasts/the-happiness-lab-with-dr-laurie-santos/reset-your-relationship-with-negative-emotions-in-2022

Tan, T.Y., Wachsmuth, L. & Tugade, M.M., 'Emotional Nuance: Examining Positive Emotional Granularity and Well-Being', *Frontiers in Psychology*, 2022

Watt Smith, Tiffany, *The Book of Human Emotions: An Encyclopedia of Feeling from Anger to Wanderlust*, Wellcome Collection, 2016

http://atlasofemotions.org

Willcox, G., 'The Feeling Wheel: A Tool for Expanding Awareness of Emotions and Increasing Spontaneity and Intimacy', *Transactional Analysis Journal*, 12(4), 274–276, 1982

Dr. Laurie Santos' podcast, The Happiness Lab, with Susan David's lighthouse analogy: www.pushkin.fm/podcasts/the-happiness-lab-with-dr-laurie-santos/emotions-are-data-so-listen-to-them

Chapter 4: **Feel-Good Emotions**
Reading, Suzy, *Rest to Reset: The busy person's guide to pausing with purpose*, Aster, 2023

Dr Kirsten Neff's webpage on compassion: https://self-compassion.org

Luo, Yangmei, Chen, Xuhai, Senqing, Qi, You, Xuqun & Huang, Xiting, 'Well-being and Anticipation for Future Positive Events: Evidences from an fMRI Study', *Frontiers in Psychology*, 8, 2199, 2018

The science of awe:
https://ggsc.berkeley.edu/images/uploads/GGSC-JTF_White_Paper-Awe_FINAL.pdf

Chapter 5: **Not So Feel-Good Emotions**
Andrew Huberman's summary of panoramic vision: https://www.scientificamerican.com/article/vision-and-breathing-may-be-the-secrets-to-surviving-2020/?amp=true

Balloon analogy on Dr Chatterjee's podcast: https://drchatterjee.com/why-emotions-matter-more-than-you-think-with-professor-marc-brackett/

Bullmore, Edward, *The Inflamed Mind: A Radical New Approach to Depression*, Short Books, 2019

Russell, Helen, How to Be Sad: Everything I've Learned About Getting Happier by Being Sad, Harper One, 2022

Unal, H., 'The Role of Socialization Process in the Creation of Gender Differences in Anger', Kadın/Women 2000 (*Journal for Woman Studies*), 5(1–2), 25–41, 2004

Brown, Brené, *Daring Greatly: How the Courage to Be Vulnerable Transforms the Way We Live, Love, Parent, and Lead*, Avery, 2012

Chapter 6: **Patterns in Emotions and Behaviours**
Tara Brach's RAIN meditation: https://tarabrach.ac-page.com/rain-pdf-download

Lyubomirsky, S. & Layous, K., 'How Do Simple Positive Activities Increase Well-Being?', *Current Directions in Psychological Science*, 22(1), 57–62, 2013

Emotions: The Ride Continues
Lane, Dr. Anne, *Nurture Your Child's Emotional Intelligence: 5 Steps to Help Your Child Cope with Big Emotions and Build Resilience*, Welbeck Balance, 2022

Dr. Martha Deiros Collado's website: www.drmarthapsychologist.com/

Dr. Emma Svanberg's website: https://mumologist.com/therapy/

Acknowledgements

I've had a lot of emotions while writing this book. Thank you to the people that helped me with them:

Supported: The time, thoughts and patience of my editor Julia and Kerry from Greenfinch books

Confident: I know my work is in safe hands with Ella, Ginny, Lipfon and Katie and the Quercus teams

Contained: Fraser, Evie and Stuart

Self-doubt: My shit fm volume controls Rona & Susan. My Keith PR Team, Douglas & Wilma.

Enjoyment: Granny and Granda, Henry and William & Co on the the unusually sunny highland holiday. Happy 70th Birthdays.

Inspiration: Emma & Jenny S and Meatloaf who, if you really think about it, made this book happen.

Index

First published in Great Britain in 2023 by

Greenfinch
An imprint of Quercus Editions Ltd
Carmelite House
50 Victoria Embankment
London EC4Y 0DZ

An Hachette UK company

A CIP catalogue record for this book is available
from the British Library

HB ISBN 978-1-52941-621-3
eBook 978-1-52941-622-0

10 9 8 7 6 5 4 3 2 1

Design by Ginny Zeal
Illustrations by Emma Hepburn

Printed and bound in Croatia by Denona

Papers used by Greenfinch are from well-managed forests and other
responsible sources.